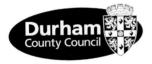

The Back
to
Basics Diet

Seven Weeks to Change Your Life

David R Hack

Matador
9 Priory Business Park,
Wistow Road, Kibworth Beauchamp,
Leicestershire. LE8 0RX
Tel: (+44) 116 279 2299
Fax: (+44) 116 279 2277
Email: books@troubador.co.uk
Web: www.troubador.co.uk/matador

ISBN 978 1783064 120

British Library Cataloguing in Publication Data.
A catalogue record for this book is available from the British Library.

Typeset in 12pt Aldine401 BT Roman by Troubador Publishing Ltd, Leicester, UK
Printed and bound in the UK by TJ International, Padstow, Cornwall

To Carol, the love of my life

Contents

Why I chose to write this book

Some years ago, I became profoundly unhappy. My father had recently died and I was struggling to cope with the aftermath of some unpleasant incidents in my business. To top it all, one day, when I was at particularly low ebb, I stood alone in front of my bedroom mirror and got the shock of my life. Somehow, I had become really fat! To make matters worse, my doctor told me I was suffering from numerous 'obesity-related' problems i.e. disruptive sleep apnea, hypertension (high blood pressure) and pre-diabetes. I was stunned. If I carried on in this way, I was headed for a lifetime of illness and an early grave. How on earth had I got myself into this state?

I grew up in a London suburb, surrounded by a loving family. My sister and I were fortunate that our parents had lived abroad before they were married (my father in India and my mother in France and Italy), meaning they both had experience of 'exotic' cuisines. As a result, we benefited from delicious, healthy meals cooked by our mum, who like many woman of that era had grown up during the war and so was adept at 'making ends meet' and using leftovers. These meals included wonderful curries (thanks, Dad) and 'Mediterranean' foods inspired by the years my mother had spent in Europe. This diet helped keep me fit, healthy and slim.

Unfortunately, soon after leaving home, the wheels began

to fall off. My bachelor years were spent in the armed forces, where each day followed a familiar pattern of 'work hard, play hard'. It wasn't long before my tailored uniform soon became a bit 'snug'. This was the start of my weight problem, which peaked about the time I stood in front of the mirror, when I had reached nearly 17 stone (240 pounds), almost 50% over my ideal weight. Enough was enough!

Desperate for answers to my declining health and gripped by a severe mid-life crisis, I took myself off to university – ostensibly to 'find myself again', but really in search of the answers to my rapidly declining health. Over the next few years, I learned about human biology, biochemistry, anatomy and human evolution before the answer I had been searching for started to emerge. In fact, it wasn't long before I realised that the solution to my ever-increasing waistline was staring me in the face. That was the start of my journey back to an ideal weight, to improved health and to a sense of happiness and contentment – a feeling I hadn't experienced for many years. What had I found? I had discovered how you and I are *designed* to eat.

We have all been led a merry dance towards a lifetime of obesity and ill health by the very foods we put in our mouths each and every day. It is time to change that now, once and for all. In fact, we need to look at our diet and lifestyle from a completely new perspective, which is what this book is all about.

I sincerely hope the Back to Basics diet will change your life, for better and forever.

David, Cumbria, September 2013

Introduction

Better a diamond with a flaw than a pebble without
– Confucius

There is little doubt that we are living in the midst of an obesity epidemic[1]. Across the globe, levels of obesity have never been higher and as a species, we are fatter now than at any time in human history[2]. As a result, we suffer from so many weight-related illnesses (e.g. type 2 diabetes) that our healthcare systems have reached breaking point. How and why have we got ourselves into this situation?

Do we really have an obesity problem?

If you or I walked down a typical high street fifty years ago, we would have struggled to spot a 'fat' person amongst the crowd. If we repeated that exercise today, we would probably find the majority of people in the crowd to be technically overweight or obese[3]. What has changed in those fifty years? Has something gone terribly wrong with our relationship with food or are we just seeing 'evolution in action', as we adapt to the foods of our highly industrialised society?

When you visit your doctor for a check-up, he or she will compare your weight against a scale known as the 'Body

Mass Index' ('BMI') – a mathematical relationship that relates your weight to your height. In the UK, the National Health Service (NHS) uses the BMI score as follows:

BMI (KG/M^2)	Description
Less than 18.5	Underweight
18.5 to less than 25	Normal
25 to less than 30	Overweight
30 or more	Obese
40 or more	Morbidly obese

By using this method, the NHS calculated that almost 25% of adults in the UK were 'obese' and 66% of men and 57% of women officially 'overweight' in 2010 [4]. The figures will almost certainly be higher by now[5].

Obesity – a worldwide problem

We certainly have an obesity problem in the UK but things are much worse in the USA, which can lay dubious claim to being the home of obesity. A couple of years ago, roughly 35% of all Americans were classed as 'clinically obese'[6].

However, if things continue as they are, *all* adults in the US will be obese by 2048[7].

The problem is not just confined to the USA – across the globe, obesity rates are skyrocketing. But does any of this really matter? I mean, isn't our body shape our business? Unfortunately not – ask any doctor and he or she will give you many reasons why carrying excess weight is bad for your health. Obesity is a leading cause of type 2 diabetes and heart disease, with at least six different types of cancer directly linked to excess body fat[8]. In fact, the link between type 2 diabetes and obesity is now *so* well established that many doctors use the phrase 'diabesity' to refer to these two interlinked conditions[9].

There are also many social problems linked to being 'big'. Obesity often leads to depression and has been linked to an increase in dementia, while obese people are often the butt of cruel jokes and can suffer from significant prejudice both socially and at work. Treating obesity is also hugely expensive – the cost could reach almost £50 billion per annum by 2050 in the UK alone.[10]

Isn't obesity just a disease of the wealthy?

For much of human history, obesity has been regarded as a 'disease of affluence'. In other words, only the wealthy could afford to eat enough to get fat. This makes sense when we consider that life was hard in the 'old days' and only the rich and powerful had access to surplus food. The peasants had to fight every day just to get enough to eat to stay alive. In fact, obesity was rare until the Industrial Revolution, when people moved en masse into the towns and cities in search of a better life. Higher wages, easier access to convenience foods and less manual labour led to increased levels of obesity amongst the new urban population. Even so, high rates of obesity were still a rare occurrence until recently.

Obesity is now mostly a disease of poverty

Recent data published by the NHS tends to support the idea that obesity is nowadays linked to poverty, at least in the UK[11]. However, in the 'richest nation on Earth' (the USA), obesity is firmly established as a disease of poverty.[12] There are numerous, complex reasons for this which are outside the scope of this book, but sadly, it is often the poorest sections of our society who present with the highest rates of obesity[13]. The picture is less clear in Britain but there is little doubt that the availability of high-calorie, low-nutrient 'fast' foods and drinks play a major part in the obesity epidemic, particularly amongst the younger and poorer members of our society.[15, 16, 17]

The Back to Basics Diet will help you lose weight

Obesity levels are out of control, but the government and medical profession are struggling to cope with the problem. Unfortunately, nobody can wave a 'magic wand' and rid us of our excess weight. Nevertheless, I hope that my healthy eating tips and recommended daily activity will help you return to a healthy weight and allow you to stay at that weight for the rest of your life. The Back to Basics diet simply helps you to re-establish a healthy relationship with real food, so it is easy to start and easy to stick with in the long term. This, of course, is not a diet at all – diets don't work, as we are about to see. Instead, you are going to recalibrate your life such that you will again be in tune with how you are *designed* to eat and live as a healthy human being.

The Back to Basics programme is not a fad diet

The ideas and techniques in this book are based on the work of top-class scientists and medical researchers – not gimmicks, fads or pseudoscience. By using some knowledge of human evolution, together with an understanding of certain aspects of our own internal chemistry, we can avoid having to count calories all the time or follow the latest celebrity-endorsed fad diet. Instead, by changing what and when we eat and embracing daily activity, we can finally unlock the secret of lifelong weight loss and health, once and for all.

In part one, I will 'set the scene' by explaining why we seem to put on weight so easily and why our weight is governed by both the types of food we eat and how we eat those foods in our modern world. Part two contains my recommended diet plans and lifestyle changes, which include a choice of two initial seven-week weight loss programmes, a lifelong 'Maintenance Programme', shopping advice, store cupboard ideas, structured meal plans and recipes, activity help and motivational tips and tricks.

If you have tried every diet in the book with little success, don't beat yourself up about it because you are most definitely not alone. Most of us find it impossible to lose weight effectively on traditional diets. The Back to Basics diet will look at weight loss from a different perspective; in re-establishing a healthy relationship with food and changing *what* and *when* we eat, we can lose weight easily and safely and again take charge of our own health destiny. All we need is a gentle push in the right direction and the right tools for the job – hopefully, you'll find all that here in the pages of this book.

A famous nutritionist once said, "Human nutrition isn't rocket science, you know. No, it is much, much more complicated that that!" I'm afraid he was probably telling the truth. However, don't worry, everything you need is here. We all need a plan to follow in life and I sincerely hope the Back to Basics programme will help *you* change *your* life once and for all to create a new, slimmer, healthier version of you.

PART ONE

Setting the Scene for the Back to Basics Diet

1

Fat? It's not your fault!

In this first chapter of the Back to Basics diet, we will see that:

- Our body weight is ultimately controlled by our calorie intake but it is the *type* of food we eat that causes obesity, not the *quantity* of food.

- Eating the wrong sort of food also causes imbalances in our body chemistry that can lead directly to weight gain.

- Such chemical imbalances often lead to an uncontrollable urge to eat that has nothing whatsoever to do with you being 'lazy' or a 'glutton'.

- Changing what and when we eat will rid us of our obesity and allow us to maintain a sensible weight for the rest of our lives.

- The Back to Basics diet helps you to reduce calorie consumption naturally, without you having to count calories at every meal.

Time to challenge the status quo

Why are you and I overweight? I'm sure that somewhere along the line you will have been told that your excess weight is just down to overeating, coupled to a lack of exercise. In other words, your 'calories in' from eating too much is more than your 'calories out' (usually from a lack of exercise), leading to an increase in body weight[1]. You may also have convinced yourself that your excess weight is caused by nothing more than greed and laziness. This is the reality we all face today in a world where obesity is regarded as a self-inflicted disease[2] – that *your* obesity is *your* fault.

Let's be clear - obesity *is* caused by an imbalance in our own personal calorie equation ('calories in' - 'calories out') and yes, many of us who are very overweight appear to eat excessive amounts of food. Obese people often find it hard to take exercise in a practical sense too, even if they have the inclination to do so. However, as you are about to discover, obesity is *not* caused simply by a lack of will power and 'poor' choice of lifestyle; indeed, nothing could be further from the truth.

Changing attitudes to obesity

So, let's begin to cheer ourselves up right now – it is definitely *not* your fault that you are overweight[4]. Yes, overweight is caused primarily by excess calorie consumption but it is the *types* of foods we eat today, rather than the quantity per se, that are largely responsible for our ballooning waistlines.[5] These 'modern' foods contain unnaturally high levels of calories *and* cause changes in chemical systems inside our body, such that we constantly try to store the energy from food in the form of fat. At the same time, we don't recognize the chemical signals that are desperately telling us we have eaten enough. Consequently, we *do* eat too many calories and then store much of the food we eat as fat. That's why it is ridiculous to suggest that we should all 'pull ourselves together' or 'show some backbone' or otherwise use good, old-fashioned willpower to lose weight when our food is groaning with unnecessary calories and our body chemistry is *so* damaged by our modern diet.

NEED TO KNOW

- Our modern diet makes it impossible to lose weight through 'willpower' alone.
- The foods we eat today contain unnaturally high levels of calories and disturb various chemical signals (hormones) inside our bodies, resulting in almost continuous weight gain and an uncontrollable urge to eat.
- Re-establishing a healthy relationship with real food will allow your hormone systems to return to sensitivity – you will no longer be 'swimming against the tide' of your own body chemistry.
- Eating real food and changing when you eat will allow effortless weight loss. No willpower required!

So, please, breath a big sigh of relief and accept right here, right now that being overweight is *not your fault*. Armed with that knowledge, what can you now do to address your weight problem? Well, you are going to make some real changes in your life that will return you to a healthy weight. You are going to change *what* and *when* you eat, so that you can start to put yourself back together and re-establish a healthy relationship with food.

In doing so, you will consume fewer calories and so lose weight safely and effortlessly and improve your health at the same time. You will become sensitive to chemical signals that tell you when you are full (and so won't eat too many calories at each meal) and will use your food to fuel the cells, tissues and organs of your body, rather than storing it as fat all the time. This is the essence of the Back to Basics diet – by eating real food at the appropriate times of the day, we can all naturally reduce our calorie intake *and* regain sensitivity to our body's various chemical signals. By returning to a natural, real food diet (inherently *low* in calories), we have no need dramatically to restrict portion size either. Remember, obesity is not your fault – it's all down to the types of food you used to eat in the 'bad old days'.

Weight gain has nothing to do with being 'lazy' or a 'glutton'

We do *not* get fat because we are lazy or because we wake up one morning and say "Oh, I think I'll be a glutton from now

Stressed out? Suffer from food addictions?

THE BACK TO BASICS DIET CAN HELP

Are you stressed, lonely or anxious?
Do you crave sweet or fatty foods?

- When you are stressed, your body produces a hormone called cortisol, which is directly related to obesity. High levels of cortisol increase cravings for sugar and fat.
- We must manage stress in order to lose weight and achieve lasting health and happiness. Try and improve your own peace of mind by getting outside for some fresh air. Try yoga, Tai Chi or meditation – anything to combat the effects of stress in our messed-up modern World.
- Try and control your cortisol levels by putting yourself first in the great scheme of things. Be mindful of your own health and happiness.
- The Back to Basics diet will help you control your cortisol levels by encouraging you to eat real food, to restrict your alcohol intake and to do daily activity.
- By being selfish for a while, you will be able to lose weight and take responsibility for your own health and happiness, perhaps for the first time in your life.

on." Instead, through no fault of our own, most of us who are overweight have got that way from a lifetime of eating the wrong sort of foods.[6, 7] As we now know, these 'wrong' foods lead to constant weight gain because they contain too many calories and affect our body chemistry such that we constantly try to store the energy from our food as fat. [9,10] The only way finally to break free of this 'food tyranny' is to change the *types* of food we eat. That's why the Back to Basics diet will help you re-establish a healthy relationship with real food by changing *what* and *when* you eat. You will then be well on your way to reversing the years of damage caused by our modern, unnatural diet.

It's all about hormones

Everything hinges on *hormones*. Most of the chemical signals sent haywire by our modern diet are hormones of one sort or another. When we change the way our bodies react to these hormones through the types of food we eat, it is very hard to avoid putting on weight, even if we try to count calories and/or use huge amounts of willpower to eat less food. Similarly, we will never lose weight in the long term by eating small portions of modern, processed foods (the basis for most diets). As we all know, it is impossible to stick to such restrictive diets for long before we 'fall off the wagon'. We will look at our 'food' hormones (primarily insulin and leptin) in more detail later. However, for now, just accept that when these particular hormones are disturbed or become ineffective because of the types of food we eat, we find it very hard, if not impossible, to lose any weight. We all intuitively know that certain things in our bodies are beyond willpower to control – such as puberty, for instance. However, willpower on its own will be just as ineffective in the 'battle of our bulge' if we don't do something about our messed-up hormones too.

OBESITY AND PUBERTY – A FAMILIAR STORY?

- Imagine a ten-year-old child about to undergo puberty – could such a child resist the changes about to take place inside their body through willpower? Of course not, the idea is obviously ridiculous.
- But why? Because, as we all know, hormones drive changes during puberty, leading to the time-honoured physical development we all experience as we grow up. The changes at puberty are beyond 'willpower' to control – puberty just happens, we can't change it.
- And obesity? Well, obesity is driven by changes in hormones too. Therefore, just like puberty, we will never lose weight by trying to resist the power of our hormones through willpower alone.

Our modern diet, comprising highly processed foods, upsets these hormonal systems in such a way that we become *resistant* to the signals these hormones are trying to send. And low and behold, if we are resistant to the hormonal signal that tells us we are full and have eaten enough, we instead suffer from an uncontrollable urge to eat.

So, overeating, leading to increased calorie intake and hence weight gain, is actually caused by the *type* of food we eat. Most of us have grown up eating highly processed 'Western' foods that have inadvertently upset certain hormone systems that lead directly to weight gain. This has nothing to do with calories; this is biochemistry.

We need to return to eating real food

Throughout this book, you will see me refer frequently to the difference between 'real' food and 'processed' food. Real food is food we are *designed* to eat[11], either by evolution or by God (depending on your point of view). We will cover these 'real' foods in much greater detail later because they underpin all the dietary changes I ask you to make in part two. However, we are simply talking about the sorts of food that sustained our ancestors over hundreds of thousands of years before the invention of agriculture – mainly small amounts of organic meat, poultry, eggs, fish and lots of fruit, vegetables, salads, some tubers and nuts.

What do these foods have in common? Well, they have all the nutrients we require for a full and healthy life but contain relatively few calories. These foods form the basis of the *ideal* human diet. A diet comprising real foods will enable you to lose weight safely and easily and allow you to stay slim and as healthy as your own genetic blueprint will allow, for the rest of your life.

Processed food – the real villain of the story

Most of us live on a diet that consists almost exclusively of *processed* foods. Such processed foods (food 'processed' by the food industry) bear little resemblance to the real, natural foods we are designed to eat. A list of such foods would fill a separate book but by and large, we are referring to the products of agriculture that are turned into mass-produced food around the globe – e.g. fast food, takeaways, supermarket ready meals, sweets, crisps, snacks, fizzy drinks, white bread, white rice, pasta, processed meats and fish, and most dairy products.

What is the problem with processed food? Well, such foods tend to give us very little, if any, real nutrition, but bucket loads of calories[12]. Coupled to a lack of exercise, a diet comprising only processed food will invariably mean we consume too many calories and so will put on weight. Similarly, eating the worst examples of these processed foods means we are denying ourselves the wonderful array of nutrients contained in real food, now known to be essential for staving off numerous nasty diseases and ensuring we have a long and healthy life.

The Back to Basics Diet will give your hormones a rest

We *do* need to eat fewer calories, but this is only one part of the story. More importantly, we need to move away from a lifetime of eating processed foods and learn to embrace all the wonderful, fresh, natural foods we are designed to eat instead. In this way, our hormones will settle down and return to normal, we will naturally eat fewer calories and we will boost our health beyond all recognition.

Changing mindsets

You may, like me, go through periods when you don't really care much about your weight or the damage it is doing to your health – you may even have convinced yourself that it somehow doesn't matter. You ignore the warnings from your friends and family (let alone your doctor) and find it much easier to put your head in the sand, rather than doing something about your weight. Sometimes, you might not care that much about yourself at all. Have I touched a raw nerve? Even if you don't always think so, trust me when I tell you that you are special, you are important and you owe it to yourself and those who love you to return to a healthy weight. If I can make the necessary changes in my life to lose weight and become healthy, so can you. Then I hope, like me, you can learn to be happy again too. It is a great feeling.

So from now on, *nobody* is blaming you for being overweight. Instead, take heart from the fact that you and I have been suffering from the ultimate con for all these years: processed food. I suppose it is not entirely fair to blame the food industry for all of our ills, as they are just doing their job and trying to meet demand from a growing World population that is eager for their ever-expanding range of products. Nevertheless, we are intelligent grown-ups and need to start making our own food choices. All we need to make the correct choices is some nutritional guidance, a basic understanding of what is really happening to us when we eat certain foods and a structured plan to ease us into a new, healthier way of eating. Well, that's all here in the pages of this book. In the meantime, let's turn our attention to the diet industry and see why, ultimately, diets just don't work.

Chapter 1 summary:

- Modern processed foods contain far too many calories for little, if any nutritional benefit.

- Such foods disturb various hormones that result in almost continuous weight gain and an uncontrollable urge to eat. By contrast, a diet of *real* food allows your hormone systems to return to sensitivity, thereby allowing you to naturally control your calorie intake. Add to this daily activity and changes to *when* you eat and weight loss will become effortless. No willpower needed.

- Remember, being overweight or obese is *not your fault.*

2

Why 'diets' just don't work

It is the mark of an educated mind to entertain a thought without accepting it. - Aristotle

In this chapter, we will explore why:

- The conventional advice to 'eat less and move more' has so obviously failed.

- Traditional restriction diets allow short-term weight loss, but are impossible to stick to for life.

- If you or I eat more calories than we burn up in any given period, we will put on weight, regardless of what you might be told in numerous fad diets.

- Continuing along our current path is non-negotiable; failing to tackle our obesity once and for all will keep us on the fat person's 'conveyor belt of life', leading to illness and an early grave.

- When you embrace a return to eating *real* food, there will be far more good news than bad about your future.

Eating less and moving more

Why has the conventional advice to 'eat less and move more' so obviously failed? If losing weight was simply a matter of cutting back on a few calories and going to the gym a couple of times a week[1], surely there would be no obesity epidemic? Instead, we see skyrocketing rates of obesity – remember that if things don't change, *all* adults in the US will be obese by 2048.

If we stop to think for a moment, we can start to piece together the reasons why this well-meaning but misguided advice is largely worthless. Yes, we do need to reduce our calorie consumption and eat less food, but simply eating less modern, processed food is not the answer[2]. We are getting precious little nutrition with this type of food in the first place, so eating *less* of it simply reduces our nutrient intake even further. Reducing our portion size will allow us to eat fewer calories, but as we all know, it is impossible to stick to such restriction diets for more than a few weeks at best.

What about moving more? This is excellent advice and burning more calories through exercise will certainly help us to lose weight, provided we eat properly as well[3]. Unfortunately, many of us view exercise as something we either avoid at all costs or perhaps dabble in once or twice a week when we take the dog out for a walk or play with the kids in the garden. So, part of the ethos of the Back to Basics diet is to encourage you to get active every single day. However, for most of us, simply moving more will have little, if any, effect on reducing our obesity until we make some fundamental changes to our diet as well[4].

Did you know that the medical profession has only one *guaranteed* cure for obesity? It's called gastrointestinal surgery. This is the reality of being too big – if we can't make changes to our diet and lifestyle that enable us to take control of our own weight and health, we face the prospect of highly intrusive surgery in our not-too-distant futures. Surely there must be a better way?

Well, you will be delighted to know that there is a better way, but it involves making significant changes to *what* you eat, *when* you eat and *how* you approach daily activity. You *will* have to make some substantial changes to your lifestyle, which I will help you with in part two. Surely this is better than the surgeon's knife?

How many 'diets' have you tried?

You don't need me to tell you that the diet industry is full of contradictions. It's no wonder we are all so confused about which diet to follow when we are faced with a constant barrage of dietary advice, such as eat 'Low-fat, high-carb' or 'high-carb, low-fat' or 'no fat at all,' 'low-carb' or 'no carb' – what on earth are we supposed to eat?

Are carbs good or bad? Should we eat more or less protein? What about fat? If it's any comfort, the scientists and medical professionals are often confused as well. [5] So, let's begin by stripping everything back to basics and see if we can work out why most diets simply don't work.

We canna change the laws of physics, Captain!

Unfortunately, we humans are just a very small part of all the living and non-living elements that make up our known Universe. Whether we like it or not, we are all governed by those ghastly 'Laws of Physics' that made life so difficult for us at school. Some of these Laws relate to whether or not we put on weight, including the Law which states that 'energy can neither be created nor destroyed' and the Law which states that the amount of energy we are able to store in our bodies as fat is equal to the amount of energy in the food we eat *minus* the energy used doing work or otherwise lost to the Universe as something called 'entropy' (heat). No more physics, I promise!

In terms of our weight, it means that:

**CHANGE IN BODY FAT =
ENERGY CONSUMED – ENERGY BURNT**
(Calories in)   (Calories out)

The experts argue endlessly over whether or not these particular Laws apply to us at all, particularly in terms of our ability to lose or put on weight[6] (I think they probably do). Some researchers believe that a 'calorie is not a calorie' and claim that it takes more energy (meaning more calories) to digest dietary protein compared to, for

17

example, carbohydrate[7]. It can all get very complicated, but as far as we are concerned, there is no getting away from the fact that if we eat more calories than we burn in any given period, we will put on weight[8]. Calorie consumption is *the* over-arching factor in all discussions about weight loss. Nevertheless, the secret to losing weight and becoming slim and healthy for the rest of our lives involves changes to our diet and lifestyle that are easy to do, but go *much* further than simply eating less and moving more.

Why dieting is not the answer

If losing weight was simply a question of eating fewer calories than we burn, why aren't we all slim? [9] Millions of people take up a new diet each year, only to fall off the wagon a few weeks later even if they have lost some weight in the meantime. The reason diets can never work in the long term is because we get hungry. If we try to lose weight on a diet of modern foods, we need to eat *tiny* portions in order to restrict our calorie intake. Yes, of course this means we are eating fewer calories, but such food restriction makes it impossible to stick to the diet in question for very long before the constant hunger becomes unbearable. Eventually, we can't stand it any more and break our diet in spectacular fashion by reaching for the nearest cream cake. Sound familiar?

Traditional diets also risk us eventually succumbing to

malnutrition. A diet entirely comprising processed foods (but in tiny portions) runs the risk of reducing the amount of nutrients we eat to dangerously low levels[10]. Any form of restriction diet, by its very nature, is liable to lead to inadequate nutrition, even if it is effective in achieving short-term weight loss. Add the fact that most of us who eat a typical 'Western' diet are not getting enough life-enhancing nutrients in the first place and we are in a whole heap of trouble! [11]

We can do much better, so in the Back to Basics diet we are going to approach the idea of calorie restriction and healthy eating in a completely new way. By replacing modern, processed foods with plentiful, healthy, real food and eating at the *right time of day* (when our body is naturally primed to use that food for fuel, rather than storing it as fat), we will naturally eat fewer calories and our portion sizes will be quite normal, so we won't get hungry. This way, we can lose weight effortlessly without resorting to willpower *and* give our health a huge boost at the same time. It's a win-win situation!

Do calories really matter?

This book is mostly going to contain lots of good news — good news about how you can change your life by losing weight and good news about how you can easily embrace a new, healthy lifestyle. In fact, I hope to inspire you to make changes in your life that will make you a much happier person all round. Nevertheless, there is inevitably going to be a bit of bad news along the way, so let's get that out of the way first. Are you sitting down? Do you have your hankie at the ready? OK, let's do the bad news right now:

If you or I eat more calories (the energy content of food) than we burn in any given time period, we will put on weight.[12]

"But Dave," I hear you say, "calories are 'old hat', an outdated concept, no longer important in the diet industry, boring and unimportant if we don't eat carbs or if we don't eat fat." Sorry, can't help you there. Eating too many calories will lead to weight gain. That is an undeniable truth, I'm afraid.

However, there is yet more good news. The Back to Basics diet will show you how to change your lifestyle and the way you eat so that you can easily bring your personal calorie equation into balance. In other words, we *do* have to eat fewer calories than we burn up, but if we eat the right type of food at the right time of day, calorie consumption will look after itself. You do *not* need to count calories specifically, unless you particularly want to use a scientific approach to your weight loss (see the Basal Metabolic Rate (BMR) sums in Appendix 1). The recommended meal plans, daily activity suggestion and tips and tricks in part two will help you get your calorie intake under control naturally, without you having to count calories ever again.

Weight loss and health – a complete package

I want you to imagine we are sneaking a look inside a secret food lab, where a volunteer has just arrived for her dietary experiment. Our volunteer is a 40-year-old lady who is 5 feet 5 inches tall and weighs 200lbs (14.3 stones). If we were to get technical and use the BMR sums in the Appendix, we would discover that she has to eat approximately 2000 calories each day to sustain her normal life. In other words, by eating 2000 calories a day and *not* changing her lifestyle, she will neither gain nor lose weight. So, to lose weight, our volunteer needs to eat *slightly fewer* calories each day and/or burn *more* calories.

Back in the secret lab, our volunteer is offered the choice of one of two sets of meals (breakfast, lunch, dinner) for the day, both of which contain the same number of calories. In other words, it doesn't matter whether she chooses to eat her meals from the first group (Group A) or the second group (Group B) – both groups contain equal calories. However, before she gets to choose her meals, she is invited outside for about an hour for a brisk walk, a short bike ride and some stretches and exercises in the garden, all of which uses up about 600 calories. On her return, she showers and dresses, now pleasantly hungry and ready for the first meal of the day. Sitting down at the table, she surveys her meal choices as follows:

Group 'A' meals:

Breakfast Two poached eggs, one round of wholemeal toast, fresh fruit, tea or coffee	**Total calories** **2000**
Lunch Grilled fish with large salad, vinaigrette dressing, fresh fruit to follow	
Dinner Sirloin steak with field mushrooms, large side salad and steamed broccoli, one glass of Cabernet Sauvignon	

Group 'B' meals:

Breakfast A two-ounce slice of chocolate cake and large dollop of vanilla ice cream	**Total calories** **2000**
Lunch A two-ounce slice of chocolate cake and large dollop of vanilla ice cream	
Dinner A two-ounce slice of chocolate cake and large dollop of vanilla ice cream	

Have I made you sit up and think? Will our volunteer lose weight on either meal group? Technically, yes. Both meal plans contain 2000 calories, so she will be in a negative calorie balance of 600 calories for either group (her BMR is 2000 calories plus 600 calories from exercise – 2000 calories from three meals today = minus 600 calories). Would she be hungry if she lived on Group B meals for any length of time? Yes. And would she be healthy if she lived on the Group B meals for weeks on end and nothing else? No!

We can't live on chocolate cake alone!

No one can live on tiny portions of chocolate cake and ice cream for very long. So, I want you to consider two separate concepts in terms of weight loss and health. They are independent ideas, but will need to be bundled together into a holistic package of dietary and lifestyle changes by the time we are through. Let's think of our journey to becoming a slimmer, healthier person (Fig 1) under two headings:

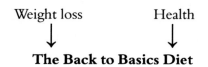

Weight loss   Health
↓   ↓
The Back to Basics Diet

Fig 1: The holistic approach to the Back to Basics diet

Although some may argue this point, the vast majority of diets only address the issue of weight loss (i.e. calorie restriction). Some diets claim to do both, but in reality very few diets succeed in effectively combining calorie restriction *and* healthy eating over the long term. As we have seen in my somewhat flippant example, calorie restriction on its own is easy (witness the three meals of tiny portions of chocolate cake and ice cream in Group B). However, simply reducing calories in isolation is doomed to failure – losing weight while contracting scurvy is not the answer!

Calorie restriction, in isolation, is not enough

Most diets fail because we are asked to dramatically restrict portion size in order to reduce calories.[13] Yes, we will lose weight in the short term, but we are unable to sustain the diet for more than a few weeks because we get hungry. Our genes are programmed to avoid starvation at all costs – if we starve ourselves, our BMR will reduce and the hormonal signals that tell us to eat will start to bellow and we will fall off our diet. Guaranteed. Happened to you? It has certainly happened to me.

So to lose weight, we *do* need to eat fewer calories, but simply reducing portion size without addressing the types of food we eat is never going to work. Any fool can design a diet that involves eating fewer calories – witness the chocolate cake and ice cream example. However, unless we combine calorie reduction with eating the right *type* of foods, we are on a hiding to nothing. Living healthily, while steadily losing weight, is more important than jumping from one fad diet to another in the vain hope of finding that 'magic wand' that will somehow return us to the image of how we thought we looked in our youth. Believe me, I've been there and it doesn't work.

I know many of you would dearly love to forget all about calories and concentrate instead on new recipes, exotic foods and diet plans? Don't worry, that's all coming in part two, where we will put together an effective weight loss plan, complete with some simple and exciting new recipes that will naturally reduce your calorie consumption as you rediscover the wonders of real, wholesome and tasty food.

Why do we really need to lose weight?

Do you want to lose weight to improve your image and fit into some lovely new clothes? Perhaps even venture onto the beach again? Well, that's fine, but there is a far more important reason why you need to get to grips with your weight. This is the last bit of bad news we are going to discuss, so keep the hankie ready:

- If you or I continue to live as we are (i.e. eating the way we have always eaten and refraining from some sort of regular exercise), our obesity will simply get worse. We will remain on the obese person's 'conveyor belt of life', leading to metabolic syndrome, then pre-diabetes, then quite probably type 2 diabetes, followed by all sorts of other nasty medical problems. Ultimately, we will be heading for an early grave.

It is time to get off the 'conveyor belt'. By following the advice in this book, you will reduce the chance of any health-related bad news at all. Unfortunately, our genes control us all, so some of us will be programmed for a difficult old age whether we like it or not. Nevertheless, we can make a huge difference to our health and to the quality of life our genes have planned for us by losing weight and getting to grips with a new, healthy lifestyle.

The Back to Basics Diet is all about good news!

This book is not a diet as such (because diets don't work), but a structured programme to help you re-establish a natural, healthy relationship with food. From now on, let's forget all about starvation, fad diets and tiny portions of chocolate cake – this is not the way to lose weight. Instead, we need to return to eating *real* food, so that we naturally reduce our calorie intake and lose weight, while giving ourselves a massive boost of healthy nutrients at the same time.

There is little doubt that our modern 'Western' diet, full of sugar and 'bad' fats, is the root cause of the current obesity epidemic. Without giving us more than a smidgen of nutritional benefit, the highly processed foods that make up the bulk of our diet not only make us fat, but also increase our risk of developing serious diseases – diabetes, heart disease, stroke, cancer etc. However, if we can grasp the nettle and strip processed foods from our diet, most of the causes of obesity will be removed in one fell swoop.

By learning to eat only real, unprocessed food, several issues resolve themselves straightaway. We will automatically consume fewer calories. We will no longer try to constantly lay down fat for a rainy day and will recognise when we have eaten sufficient food. Finally, our cravings for sugar will ease and we will naturally stabilise our blood sugar levels without having to eat something every five minutes.

Fat? Remember, it's not your fault!

Let's finish this chapter by reminding ourselves of what we discussed right at the beginning of the book – it is *not your fault* that you are overweight or obese. Yes, many of us eat too much and put on weight; however, this is due to the foods in our modern diet disturbing our body chemistry in a way that makes it impossible for us to stop overeating. Most of us are overweight because we have spent a lifetime eating the wrong sort of foods; not only have we consumed too many calories for little, if any, nutritional benefit, we have also sent our internal weight 'regulating systems' haywire, leading to steady and continual weight gain.

So, I don't want you to go on a diet, but instead change your diet to one we are *designed* to eat. The time has come to move away from fad and yo-yo dieting by embracing a new way of life, involving sensible, healthy eating and long-term weight loss, just as Nature intended.

Moving on

To find out why our modern diet is *so* damaging to our health, we need to go right back to the beginning. By looking at the *original* human diet, we can start to unlock the dietary secrets that will rid us of our obesity and allow us to stay at our correct weight for the rest of our lives. This means we have to go on a journey to a world of wild animals and even wilder people. We need to go back in time to the depths of the African continent, where the human race first appeared, to see how a 'hunter-gatherer' lifestyle allowed our earliest ancestors to live healthy lives, free of most of our modern diseases.

Having finally moved 'Out of Africa' to colonise every corner of the planet, these early ancestors paved the way for the much later appearance of anatomically 'modern' humans a few hundred thousand years ago. And do you know what? In terms of what they needed to eat to keep them at the very peak of their powers, these early humans were *identical* to a much more modern version of a human such as you or I.

Chapter 2 summary:

- Simply eating less and moving more will not work if we continue to eat modern, processed foods. That is the reason why traditional 'restriction' diets may enable short-term weight loss, but are impossible to stick to for life.

- If you or I eat more calories than we burn in any given period, we will put on weight, regardless of what you might be told in numerous fad diets.

- Failing to tackle our obesity once and for all will keep us on the fat person's 'conveyor belt of life', leading to illness and an early grave.

- When you embrace a return to eating real food, there will be far more good news than bad about your future!

3

Our 'Hunter-Gatherer' origins

*Mankind differs from the animals only by a little and most people
throw that away*
- Confucius

In this chapter, we will discover that:

- Evolution, through natural selection, has led to an exquisitely-designed creature called a human being.

- We abuse this remarkable creature everyday by feeding it foods it is not designed to eat.

- Our modern diet, full of sugar and processed food, is completely out of kilter with the foods our ancestors ate for hundreds of thousands of years.

- Our body chemistry, which is directly responsible for governing whether or not we lose or gain weight, developed over millennia as our ancestors evolved into people like us, i.e. modern day humans.

- This process of evolution (over millennia) occurred

across the globe under a virtually identical, natural human diet.

* The invention of agriculture, at first sight such a huge boon to the success of the human race, actually marked the beginning of the slippery slope towards the obesity and ill health we see all around us today.

Evolution holds the key

The opening lecture of my biology degree began with a slide containing the following quote:

"Nothing in Biology Makes Sense Except in the Light of Evolution"
(Theodosius Dobzhansky; 1973)

As Charles Darwin discovered all those years ago, the process of evolution by natural selection underpins the entire natural world. Darwin worked with plants and animals, but his ideas are equally relevant to our origins as human beings.

A very remarkable mammal

Millions of years of evolution, via natural selection, has led to a remarkably successful and intelligent mammal called a human being. I like to think of us as exquisitely-designed biological machines, certainly in terms of how we control our weight. However, many of us abuse this wonderful machine we call our body by eating foods we are *not* designed to eat[1].

By delving into the story of human evolution, we can begin to uncover the reasons *why* we put on weight so easily, why we are most certainly *not* adapted to our current Western diet and why the great scholar Professor Jared Diamond (*The Third Chimpanzee: The Evolution and Future of the Human Animal* and *Guns, Germs, and Steel: The Fates of Human Societies*) described the invention of agriculture as "the worst mistake in the history of the human race."[2] By looking back at our earliest history on this planet and learning about the original human diet, we can start to make changes to *our* diet and lifestyle that will return us to a normal weight. In turn, this will help us live the longest and healthiest lives that our particular genetic 'throw of the dice' will allow.

Our modern diet is making us ill

Our modern diet is so out of kilter with how we are designed to eat that we are literally poisoning ourselves with the foods we eat.[3] If we are to have any chance of finally getting to grips with our obesity, we simply must understand why eating the way we do today is so at odds with how we are *supposed* to eat. So let's find out what we should be eating by setting off on a journey back through our evolutionary past to the dawn of time, when our ancestors, the early primates, ran wild and free across the Earth.

The story of 'us'

Our story begins about 65 million years ago (mya). This was when the earliest apes first started to appear in North America before emigrating to Africa to become the forerunner of all current living primates, including humans (Fig 2).

We can trace our origins all the way back to these early apes. Our more recent ancestors are called the *Hominids*, creatures who developed from the earlier primates and appeared on Earth about 15 mya. These very early prototype humans had large brains and were able to walk upright. However, it wasn't until much later (about 200,000 years ago) that we 'anatomically modern humans' first made our entrance onto the stage of evolutionary history[4]. None of this happened

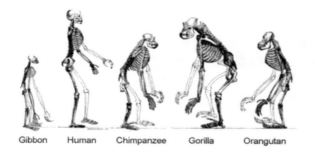

Gibbon   Human   Chimpanzee   Gorilla   Orangutan

Fig 2. The Third Chimpanzee? Our similarity to the Great Apes is clear from a comparison of primate skeletons (image courtesy of Wikipedia).

overnight; it took millions of years of evolution and natural selection before modern humans finally emerged on the scene, with many intermediate steps along the way.[5]

Australopithecus – our (very) early ancestors!

One of the first prototype human groups ('genus' in science speak) was called *Australopithecus*.[6] The *Australopiths* had brains about 35% the size of ours and stood just 4 feet tall, but were quite a successful group. They walked upright, which was the first evidence of *bi-pedalism* in our ancestry. No one is quite sure why we started walking on our hind legs, but the academics are convinced this ability to walk probably played a major role in the later development of our large human brains.

The original Back to Basics Diet

So, what did the *Australopiths* eat? By looking at the patterns of wear on *Australopith* fossil teeth, scientists have worked out that our earliest ancestors ate a diet almost exclusively consisting of fruit, vegetables and tubers; some of the more robust *Australopithecus* species also ate nuts and seeds – a few ate animal flesh, too.

Australopithecus probably died out about 2 mya. Not all living creatures prove successful in the long term, but that's evolution for you. So, what came next? Well, as far as we can tell, the next 'prototype humans' to appear were species of the genus *Homo*. Today, humans (*Homo sapiens*) are the last surviving species of this genus, but in the past there were a number of *Homo* species – some of which were directly involved in the development of modern humans.

Out of Africa

There are essentially two different opinions as to what happened next. Either we modern humans evolved separately in Africa (about 250, 000 years ago) and then spread out to replace all the original *Homo* populations or we arose independently from various earlier *Homo* populations already spread across the globe.[8, 9] Regardless of which is correct, 'anatomically modern humans' appeared on planet Earth about 200, 000 years ago.

So, what did the early *Homo* species eat? Well, it seems they ate pretty much what the *Australopiths* ate, but with the addition of wild meat and fish.[10] Did any of these ancestral human species suffer from our modern 'diseases of civilisation'? Not as far as we can tell – as yet, no one has found any significant evidence of heart disease or cancers in the archaeology of these early humans[11].

The 'Hunter-Gatherer' diet

So, we know that we evolved from a plant-eating ancestor, via *Australopithecus* etc. Nevertheless, at some point, our ancestors discovered the benefits of eating meat. After the discovery of 'Lucy', the skeleton of an early species of

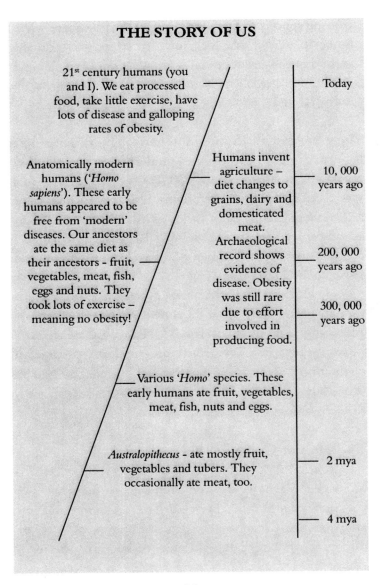

THE STORY OF US

21st century humans (you and I). We eat processed food, take little exercise, have lots of disease and galloping rates of obesity.

Today

Anatomically modern humans ('*Homo sapiens*'). These early humans appeared to be free from 'modern' diseases. Our ancestors ate the same diet as their ancestors - fruit, vegetables, meat, fish, eggs and nuts. They took lots of exercise – meaning no obesity!

Humans invent agriculture – diet changes to grains, dairy and domesticated meat. Archaeological record shows evidence of disease. Obesity was still rare due to effort involved in producing food.

10, 000 years ago

200, 000 years ago

300, 000 years ago

Various '*Homo*' species. These early humans ate fruit, vegetables, meat, fish, nuts and eggs.

Australopithecus - ate mostly fruit, vegetables and tubers. They occasionally ate meat, too.

2 mya

4 mya

Australopithecus that may have used stone tools to cut meat off animal bones almost 3.5 mya, it appears we became carnivores much earlier than first thought.[20]

It seems, then, that we humans gave up a completely vegetarian lifestyle millions, rather than thousands, of years ago. Nevertheless, for millions of years until the advent of agriculture about 10, 000 years ago (less than the 'blink of an eye' in evolutionary terms), all humans evolved on a diet of basically the same food. What did our ancestors eat over this enormous period of time? There were no shops, no takeaways and no restaurants, so all food was wild and had to be gathered (wild fruits and vegetables) or hunted or scavenged (meat, fish, eggs etc). Although the specifics varied across the globe, many features of the ancestral diet were remarkably consistent:

- A complete lack of processed food.
- Not much grain.
- No dairy (have you tried to milk a wild animal?)
- Virtually no sugar.
- No modern man-made fats (fats were eaten with relish, but prehistoric wild animals were lean by modern standards and contained healthy, natural fats).

The secret is in the shape of our gut!

It may come as a surprise to learn that in many ways we are designed to eat a similar diet to that of the chimpanzee.

Believe it or not, we share about 98.4% of our DNA with chimps; in terms of our ideal diet, we are even closer than that.

Everything hinges on the size and shape of our colon! Both humans and chimps have a sacculated (or 'haustrated') colon, a sure sign that we are derived from a plant-eating ancestor.[12] Similarly, neither humans nor chimps can synthesise Vitamin C, which is best obtained from fruits and vegetables in the diet. Taken together these two aspects of our digestion clearly point to the fact that we are descended from a plant-eating ancestor.

Humans are not chimpanzees

However, we are *not* designed to eat the same diet as a chimpanzee. Chimps have much bigger colons than we do, whereas we have more of our gut as small intestine. Chimps eat lots of tough plant material, but due to their huge colons, they can break this plant food down slowly by fermentation. Chimps do eat some meat as well, but by contrast, we have become adapted to a high-quality diet of fruits, vegetables and animal foods (lean, organic meats and fish). Both apes and humans are unusual in the length of time it takes for food to transit through the body compared, say, to a carnivore (it takes roughly forty-five hours for high-fibre food to transit our guts, whereas a polar bear will poop out the remains of his seal dinner in about seventeen hours).[13] This is important in terms of our weight loss, as we will see later on.

Our recent ancestors ate a perfect diet

Wild chimps don't seem to suffer from obesity or 'diseases of civilisation' and neither did our ancient ancestors, as far as we can tell from the archaeological record. If we 'dig' a bit deeper, we also find an absence of obesity and modern diseases in many contemporary hunter-gatherer societies and in people

THE DESIGN OF OUR GUT SHOWS US THE WAY TO OUR PERFECT DIET

- The shape of our colon shows we are descended from a plant-eating ancestor – we are designed to eat fruits and vegetables.
- We can't make Vitamin C, so we are supposed to get this micronutrient from the fruit and vegetables in our diet.
- The differences in our gut design, compared to chimps, shows we are meant to eat a high-quality diet of fruit and vegetables, 'topped off' with meats and fish.
- Our guts have a limited capacity because we are designed to eat a predominantly vegetarian diet. This means we are supposed to 'fill up' with healthy, low-calorie, nutrient rich plant food, which takes a while to digest and so stops us from otherwise eating too many calories (from, for example, junk food). Add some legumes, a few nuts, and some (organic) meat or fish to our diet, and we end up very close to the diet that evolution has spent millions of years perfecting.

whom until recently maintained a traditional lifestyle – for example, farmers in Crete up until the 1970s. [14,15]

What can we learn from these healthy people? Well, they took a lot of exercise and so used up a lot of calories every day. They ate food that was naturally *low* in calories but *high* in nutrients (a mostly vegetarian diet, with meat or fish on high days and holidays). So, just like their ancestors, the original human 'hunter-gatherer' diet was predominantly vegetarian, with opportunistic meat-eating now and again (hunting is actually quite difficult – more difficult than first thought). And due to the slow passage of food through the human gut, our ancestors could fill up on plant food (so meeting their needs for energy) and make use of infrequent meals of animal protein and fats to add high-quality nutrients to their diet. This is much more efficient than your average chimp, who has to eat vastly *more* plant food in order to gain a complete array of nutrients.

Agriculture – the biggest mistake in human history?

Unfortunately, everything went a bit south about 10, 000 years ago when the human race invented agriculture. At first glance, this seems like a huge leap forward in the evolution of man, as for first time food availability could be pretty much guaranteed. Indeed, by growing crops and raising livestock, these early farmers were able to break the seasonal cycle of 'feast or famine' common to all hunter-gatherer societies. So, this must have been a huge step forward for the human race, right?

Not necessarily. The skeletal remains of the early agriculturists appear to be shorter, misshapen with disease and obviously much less healthy than skeletons found in the fossil record from any number of earlier hunter-gatherer communities.[16] Perhaps this was why Jared Diamond called the invention of agriculture "the biggest mistake in human history?" OK, he was talking mostly about sociological issues, but something obviously went badly awry with the human diet when, as a species, we decided to abandon our evolutionary past as hunters and adopt the plough instead. Ironically, the problem stems from something to do with plants.

Plants want to survive, too

Just like all other life on Earth, plants are subject to the forces of evolution and so exist primarily for one reason: to pass on their genes.[17] Plants have been around a long time and although they appear at first glance to be less sophisticated than animals and humans, the pressures of natural selection have led to remarkable strategies in plants to help them pass on their genes successfully.

Plants have a tough life. They have to compete with their neighbours for nutrients and water from the soil and have to fight for access to sunlight, so they can grow and store energy through photosynthesis. Meanwhile, they have to deal with passing animals that take great delight in eating their leaves and stems for lunch.

Now, think about this for a moment: if you are a

successful plant, which part of your anatomy do you *not* want the passing rabbit to eat? How do plants pass on their genes? Of course, plants have seeds containing the genetic information ready for the next generation. Many plants encase their seeds in highly nutritious and colourful fruits, which they are more than happy for the passing mammal to eat. This way, the seeds will pass through the digestive tract of the animal in question and be deposited somewhere else in the forest, so spreading the genes of this particular plant species far and wide. That's evolution in action! However, the plant does *not* want its seeds eaten and destroyed. Consequently, many plants have evolved numerous cunning ways to make their seeds unpalatable (or often, downright poisonous) to animal grazers. As an example, let's look at a fairly well-known plant called wheat.

Wheat – a double-edged sword

Eating wheat (our daily bread?) in many ways defines us as a Western society. However, which part of the wheat plant do we actually eat? We grind up the wheat grain to make flour, which as we all know is then used to make bread and lots of other gooey, sticky delights, but have you ever stopped to think what a wheat grain actually is?

Technically it's a combination of a fruit and a seed, but as far as we are concerned, the grain of the wheat plant is the seed of wheat. Wheat seeds (grains) have been at the heart of the Western diet for thousands of years, proving to be nutritious and an ideal food source in the early days of agriculture. However, do you think wheat is a *natural* human food?

Gluten and lectin – two reasons to give wheat a wide berth

The wheat seed contains substances (such as gluten and lectin) that turn out to be rather nasty when consumed by humans.[18] Gluten is used by grass-type plants, like wheat, as a food source in the seed for the new plant embryo during germination. Lectins are proteins that can bind to various sugars in cells and then help out with lots of complex cellular tasks. So these two substances, gluten and lectin, are designed by evolution to help wheat-type plants (and rye, barley etc) pass on their genes. However, this doesn't mean we are designed to eat wheat seeds ourselves.

What is the problem with eating gluten and lectin? They are proteins after all, so must provide us with some of our daily protein requirement? Yes and no. Yes, they provide us with a source of protein, but they also make us ill and are now known to be a major cause of the obesity epidemic we see all around us.

Our 'Hunter-Gatherer' ancestors point the way to a perfect diet

For the majority of human history, mankind existed in tribes and communities around the World that lived in a similar

THE PROBLEM OF WHEAT

- We eat the seeds of the wheat plant in the form of flour.
- Like all plants, wheat wants to *protect* its seeds at all costs.
- The wheat plant has evolved some unpleasant chemicals (particularly gluten and lectin) that are mainly designed to do other tasks but happen to make the seeds of the wheat plant unpalatable.
- The chemicals in the seeds of a wheat plant means that wheat flour is most definitely *not* a natural human food.
- Processed (white) bread provides too many calories for only a modicum of nutrition, is directly linked to the causes of obesity and can lead to potentially life-threatening illness and disease.
- Fancy that sandwich now?

way.[19] Even though the content of the diet varied due to geography, *all* foods eaten prior to the invention of agriculture were real, unprocessed foods (vegetables, fruit, meat, naturally-occurring fats, poultry, fish, nuts and eggs). By happy coincidence, such unprocessed food is fairly low in calories, too.

Unprocessed food does not, generally, lead to inflammation in the body. Unprocessed food is full of natural and healthy proteins, fats and carbohydrates, plus abundant micronutrients such as minerals, vitamins and the catch-all phytonutrients – the wonderful life-giving and irreplaceable chemicals found in fruits and vegetables. As a species we are not, under any circumstances, designed to live almost exclusively on the seeds of just four plants (wheat, rice, corn and rye).

It is time to wave goodbye to baked goods!

So, we are not going to eat bread and cakes anymore, are we? Instead, just like our primate ancestors, we need to eat a predominantly vegetarian diet. That way, we can build our diet around plant food that is relatively low in calories but nutrient-rich (full of all the chemicals, vitamins, anti-oxidants, proteins, healthy fats essential for health.)

Please don't panic, this is not as bad as it sounds! A predominantly vegetarian diet still means we can enjoy our Sunday lunch, steaks, roast chicken, fresh fish, pork chops etc – it just means we are going to replace all the processed foods in our diet with real food (fresh fruits, salads and vegetables) and combine them with tasty sources of animal protein. And by filling up on vegetables, you won't need much meat, poultry or fish anyway, so will almost certainly spend less money on the Back to Basics diet than you used to spend on processed junk.

By adding legumes, a few nuts and seeds, and some organic meat or fish to our new, predominantly vegetarian diet, we end up eating in a way that evolution has spent millions of years perfecting on our behalf. Add some onions

GLUTEN AND LECTIN

(Some very good reasons why we should give
wheat a wide berth)

- Gluten (and one of its proteins called gliadin) causes inflammation of the gut in most people. It is believed that coeliac disease, a serious autoimmune condition, is caused by the body's intolerance to the gliadin protein in gluten.
- Most of us are intolerant to the effects of gluten in our diet. This leads to inflammation of the gut ('leaky gut'), where chemicals that should remain in the gut, such as the toxins from nasty bacteria, can cross into the blood stream and do damage around the body.
- Such inflammation and 'leaky gut' means our immune system makes antibodies, which can then cause untold problems elsewhere. Gliadin has a similar chemical structure to proteins in other parts of our body (e.g. in the thyroid and the pancreas), so the antibodies end up attacking these other proteins accidently.
- There is also evidence that antibodies to gluten might be implicated in both heart disease and cancer, too.
- Lectin also upsets our guts, causing inflammation and 'leaky gut'. In terms of obesity, lectin interferes with a chemical signaling system in the body that is designed to tell us we are full – so stop eating! If these signals are ignored, we don't realise we are full and keep eating. Result: we eat too many calories and get fat.

and garlic, a little olive oil perhaps, the odd glass of red wine and the company of good friends and family and we will be eating in a way that has enabled millions of people across the globe to avoid obesity and enjoy a healthy, happy life.

So, it is time to smile, time to laugh and time to raise two fingers to the old you. It is time to enjoy real food again, to buy and cook seasonal fruits and vegetables and to source healthy, organic sources of protein. From now on, I want you to forget fad diets and yo-yo dieting and instead look forward to a new way of life, involving sensible, healthy eating and long-term weight loss.

Let's now turn to food itself; what it comprises, what it is made of and why some knowledge of food science will help us understand why our modern diet is so alien to the way we are designed to eat.

Chapter 3 summary:

- Evolution, through natural selection, has led to an exquisitely-designed biological machine called a human being. This process of evolution occurred under a virtually identical, natural human diet.

- We are designed to eat a predominantly vegetarian diet, plus small amounts of organic proteins and healthy fats.

- Our modern diet, full of sugar and processed food, is completely out of kilter with the foods our ancestors ate for hundreds of thousands of years.

- By returning to our original diet, the diet we are designed to eat, we will lose weight effortlessly and see a remarkable improvement in our health, too.

- A return to a real food, original human diet, plus some daily activity, gives us the best chance of returning to health and becoming slim again, just like our ancestors before we invented agriculture and started eating sandwiches!

4

The food we eat

*'I do not like broccoli. And I haven't liked it since I was a little kid
and my mother made me eat it. And I'm
President of the United States and I'm not going
to eat any more broccoli.'*
- President George Bush

In this very important chapter, we will discover that:

- Our modern diet is making us fat because it comprises foods we are not designed to eat.

- Our health is dictated by the amount of micronutrients in our diet.

- Proteins are an essential part of the human diet. Although we derive much of our protein from eating meat and fish, we can actually satisfy all our protein needs with a balanced vegetarian diet.

- Fats have had a very bad press, when in fact they are an essential part of the natural human diet.

- Processed carbohydrate lies at the heart of the current obesity epidemic. However, carbohydrates in real food should make up the bulk of our diet.

To work out which foods we should eat and which we should avoid, we need to understand something about the chemical structure of the different sorts of food in our diet. By studying the make-up of our food in this way, we can start to see why certain foods upset our internal chemistry and make us fat. In fact, much of this food science underpins the dietary secrets explained later in the book. What follows may be a little complicated, but it is well worth making the effort to understand how our food affects us in this fundamental way. So, please treat this chapter as a reference, and dip in and out of it now and again when you need to refresh your memory.

Food – friend and foe?

Our modern diet makes us fat, mainly because it is completely out of kilter with how we are designed to eat as healthy human beings. Let me repeat that – our modern diet is making us fat because it comprises foods we are *not* designed to eat.[1] Most of us are overweight because of our love affair with high-calorie, processed foods, so if you were secretly hoping for a diet that would allow you to eat whatever foods you like, but perhaps in smaller quantities, then this book is probably not for you.

Unfortunately, if we want to lose weight safely and effectively, certain foods are going to have to go. However, once you accept that things have to change, we can look at all the really tasty, healthy food that we can eat in abundance instead.

The chemistry of life

Our bodies are extraordinarily complex and contain a baffling array of cells, tissues and organs. Literally millions of chemical reactions take place inside these cells and organs all the time, each one of which allows us to live, grow and generally exist as a healthy human being. These chemical reactions are usually referred to as human biochemistry, meaning the 'chemistry of life', and how all the biochemical reactions interplay to make us work is referred to as human physiology. We don't need any more detail than that, but you might see me refer to these terms in later chapters.

Metabolism

When we eat something, the various foodstuffs are broken down in our digestive system to their component parts. This breaking down process, known as *catabolism*, is how we obtain the building blocks for all the other chemicals and substances we have to make to keep us alive. This is one part of our overall metabolism. During catabolism, energy is released as something called 'ATP' (the petrol of our body chemistry). Later, we use these building blocks in a complementary process called *anabolism*, where new chemicals and products are built up from scratch, using the energy of ATP, as previously released during catabolism.

METABOLISM - THE TECHNICAL STUFF (OPTIONAL!)

- Metabolism is the sum of all the biochemical processes in our bodies that allow us to function as a healthy human being. There are a vast number of chemical reactions involved in metabolism but in terms of our weight, there are two key processes, known as catabolism and anabolism.
- Catabolism is the breaking down of big molecules into smaller bits, during which energy is released. Catabolism can either be the breakdown of the foods we eat at each meal or the burning of stored food (e.g. glycogen, fat) for fuel. The process of catabolism releases energy in the form of 'ATP', to drive our body chemistry. Catabolism is controlled by numerous hormones e.g. cortisol, glucagon, adrenalin.
- Anabolism is the opposite of catabolism and involves the building up of complex molecules from smaller bits (e.g. new cells and tissue, such as muscle). Anabolism requires energy (ATP) and is mediated by hormones too (e.g. the anabolic steroids and insulin).
- If catabolism exceeds anabolism, there will be an excess of energy. We store this excess as either glycogen or fat.

You may have heard of the illegal drugs used by some (misguided) athletes known as anabolic steroids. These drugs are designed to enhance the body's anabolism or build-up of cells, particularly in muscles – with obvious, if illegal, benefits.

All we really need to remember is that there are two distinct processes (catabolism and anabolism) that occur during and shortly after eating food. Much of the reason we put on weight is due to imbalances in these two biochemical systems, simply because our present way of eating is out of balance with our biochemistry.[2] Let's now look at the components of the food in our diet.

The food components of our diet

We generally talk about food under one of two main headings; *macronutrients* make up the bulk of the food we eat, while *micronutrients* are the invisible minerals and vitamins that are responsible for boosting our health and fighting disease (Fig 3).

In many ways, it is the amount of micronutrients in our diet that decides our level of health and wellbeing. However, for now, I want to concentrate on the main classes of food that we have all heard of, namely the macronutrients:

MACRONUTRIENTS	MICRONUTRIENTS
Protein	Water
Fat (Triglycerides)	Vitamins
Carbohydrates	Minerals Anti-oxidants Phytochemicals etc

Fig 3. The classification of foods by nutrient content.

Protein

Proteins are probably the most important nutrients of all and are absolutely vital to our health. We have all heard of proteins and know that they are in meat and fish, but what are they exactly?

Proteins are long-chain molecules made up from linked sub-units called *amino acids*. Complex little molecules themselves, amino acids have various chemical properties and consist of a mixture of the atoms of carbon, hydrogen, oxygen and nitrogen, in distinct arrangements depending on the amino acid in question. Amino acids can be linked up in longer and longer chains to form protein molecules. Of the twenty-two amino acids known to exist, nine are classed as essential; this means that we are unable to make these particular amino acids ourselves and so have to take them in through our diet to maintain our health.[3]

Proteins are vital to our health

As most of the important processes in our bodies rely on protein in one form or another, proteins are obviously vital to our health. The growth and renewal of our cells and organs depends on the presence of proteins, while virtually every chemical reaction that takes place inside us is controlled by a protein known as an *enzyme* – a catalyst that speeds up chemical reactions.[4] Proteins are involved in myriad other biological tasks as well. However, there is one group of proteins that we have touched on already that are at the heart of the obesity/weight loss story; these crucial proteins are called *hormones* and you will meet some of them again later.

The word *protein* conjures up images of large steaks sizzling on the barbeque, but it is largely a myth that we have to eat lots of animal food in order to get our daily protein requirements. We can easily get all the protein we need from plants, whether fruit, vegetables, nuts, seeds or legumes.[5] Nevertheless, unless you are barred from such foods on religious, ethical or moral grounds, I recommend you eat certain animal protein, such as fish, as part of your new diet. We'll talk about proteins again, but for now, let's look at the other classes of macronutrients.

Fats – a 'potted' history!

Of all the foods we eat, poor old fats have endured the worst press. OK, eating huge amounts of fat is going to make it hard

Amino acids	
Essential amino acids	**Non-essential amino acids**
Histidine	Alanine
Isoleucine	Arginine
Leucine	Asparagine
Lysine	Aspartic acid
Methionine	Cysteine
Phenylalanine	Glutamic acid
Threonine	Glycine
Tryptophan	Ornithine
Valine	Proline
	Selenocysteine
	Serine
	Taurine
	Tyrosine

to lose weight and we are certainly not designed to eat man-made fats or the fat of artificially reared, unhealthy, domesticated livestock. However, I am convinced that fats have been unfairly treated and firmly believe there is a fundamental misunderstanding about the role of fat in a healthy diet. [6]

Ancel Keys

Up until about the time of the Second World War, the most common medical treatment for obesity was a low-carbohydrate diet (eat meat and fats, but avoid the carbs). This all goes back to the Victorian era, when a rather corpulent Englishman called William Banting famously made public the story of his weight loss on just such a diet (his is an interesting story and if you want to learn more about this early form of low-carb diet, have a look at Gary Taubes's book, *Good Calories, Bad Calories*[7]).

However, things changed after the war when an American scientist named Ancel Keys claimed that high levels of saturated fat in the diet led to heart disease. Although nothing to do with obesity, this hypothesis was seized upon as 'gospel' by the US Government, which later published the famous 'eat a low-fat, high-carbohydrate diet for health' mantra – advice that has dominated the world of human nutrition for the last fifty years.[8]

Many people, me included, believe that the 'low-fat, high-carbohydrate' mantra has completely backfired, leading to the skyrocketing levels of obesity we see all around us today. Nevertheless to many of us who are trying to lose weight, 'fat' is a dirty word. There is so much confusion around this particular foodstuff that we ought to spend a few minutes getting to the bottom of the story, once and for all. So let's now have a quick and unbiased look at fats in a bit more detail.

ANCEL KEYS AND THE SEVEN COUNTRIES STUDY

Ancel Keys was a physiologist who invented a famous form of soldier's rations during World War 2. Because of this, he had the 'ear' of the US Government in respect of nutritional advice.

After the war, Keys started working in the field of diet and cardio-vascular disease; later, he published the 'Seven Countries Study', a rather controversial statistical analysis of the relationship between diet and cardio-vascular disease in men in different countries (nominally twenty-two countries, but later reduced to seven).[9]

The 'Seven Countries Study' has been criticised, largely due to Key's interpretation of the data. Nevertheless, the results of this huge project led Keys to his 'diet-heart' hypothesis, which directly influenced US Government dietary policy for a generation. This eventually resulted in the official advice to 'eat a low-fat, high-carb diet'.

Fats – a true story!

Both the fats in our diet and the fat we carry around our bodies are known as *triglycerides*. A triglyceride is a molecule that consists of a backbone of an alcohol called *glycerol* attached to three (hence 'Tri') fatty acids (Fig 4).

Please don't be alarmed by this diagram, I just want to show you what 'fat' looks like – I promise there won't be a

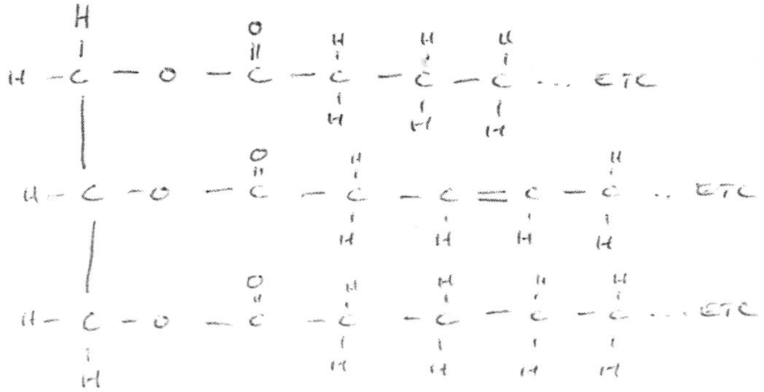

Fig 4. The component parts of a triglyceride.

test later! What do all those 'C's' and 'H's' mean? This is just chemistry shorthand for many atoms of carbon (the 'C'), joined to many atoms of hydrogen (the 'H'). Out there in the real world, carbon needs to form four chemical bonds to be stable electrically. If each carbon atom in the fatty acid chain makes all four bonds, our fat is *saturated* – which means that all the bonds of each carbon atom are complete. However, if there isn't enough hydrogen to go round, carbon can be crafty and form a double bond with an adjacent carbon atom instead, so making an *unsaturated* fat. If just one double bond is formed, the fat is said to be a *monounsaturated* fat (e.g. olive oil). If there is more than one double bond in the fatty acid chain, then the fat is referred to as *polyunsaturated* (e.g. numerous vegetable oils). So, now you know where all those strange fat names come from.

The energy in fats

What does all this organic chemistry mean? Well, any molecule that is stuffed full of hydrogen atoms, such as a saturated fat, is full of potential chemical energy. Fat is a very efficient source of energy; if you burned some in a laboratory, it would yield nine calories of heat energy per gram of weight. This is compared to most carbohydrates (i.e. sugars) that only yield four calories of heat energy per gram. Fat, therefore, is an excellent source of energy. By the way, saturated fats such as butter and lard are usually solids at room temperatures because of the bulky three-dimensional molecular shape needed to cram in all those hydrogen atoms. *Mono-* and *polyunsaturated* fats are generally liquid at room temperatures.

Saturated fats – aren't they the enemy?

There is nothing inherently wrong with saturated fats. They are part of a natural human diet, contain numerous helpful vitamins, are essential for various tasks in our body and are a highly efficient source of energy.[10] Saturated fats were hugely important in our ancestors' diet and were often the main source of calories and nutrients for Aboriginal peoples such as the Inuit and certain Plains Native Americans. [11]

Saturated fat is part of a natural human diet

Think of it this way: if saturated fat was an inherently toxic substance, do you not think that after millions of years of evolution, natural selection would have come up with a different way of storing energy inside our bodies? Apart from childbirth, which seems terribly clumsy and difficult for human females, natural selection has resulted in a stunningly efficient body plan for us humans. Why would the enormous pressure of evolutionary time have come up with fat as a means of storing food energy inside us *if* fat was toxic or otherwise dangerous to us? The answer is that real, unprocessed fat, ideally from vegetable sources or organic animals, is a perfectly natural human food. [12,13]

Getting our 'Omegas' in the right proportion

Remember I said that there were nine essential amino acids in proteins that we could only obtain through our diets? Well, there are also some essential fatty acids, and just like the proteins mentioned earlier, they cannot be made in our bodies and so must be taken in via our food. These fatty acids are vital to our health (they are used, amongst other things, to build our cell walls and manufacture hormones) and act as the building blocks of other fatty acids that we have the ability to make ourselves.[14]

The two main essential fatty acids are called *linoleic acid*, an Omega 6 fatty acid, and *alpha-linolenic acid*, an Omega 3 fatty acid. But what on earth does 'Omega 6' and 'Omega 3' mean? Well, the '6' and the '3' refer to the position of the double bond in the fatty acid chain, that's all. It seems one of the most important aspects of a healthy diet is getting these two fatty acids in the right proportion.[15] The experts argue until they are blue in the face about how much fat we should eat, so it makes sense to be careful both about the amount of fat we eat and the balance of these two essential fatty acids in our diet.

So, what is the correct ratio of Omega 6: Omega 3? Well, it seems that we evolved to eat these fats in a ratio that was pretty close to one-to-one or thereabouts.[17] This was relatively easy for our *Paleo* ancestors to achieve because the real, natural foods they ate had a balance of Omega 6: Omega 3 in the correct ratio. However, most modern, processed foods contain far too much Omega 6 but not enough Omega 3, completely upsetting that natural balance.

Basically, we need to eat more Omega 3 and less Omega 6 fatty acids. Omega 3 is found in certain plants, such as flaxseeds and also in many oily fish (e.g. mackerel, tuna, sardines). So, all we need to do to strike the correct balance between the Omega 6 fats and the Omega 3 fats in our diet is to eat less Omega 6 fats, to avoid most vegetables oils such as sunflower oil and all modified trans fats, and eat more foods containing Omega 3 oils. If we then remove sugar from our diet too, we can begin to use fat for fuel, just as evolution has designed us to do.

ESSENTIAL FATTY ACIDS
('THE OMEGAS')

- *Linoleic acid* is an unsaturated, essential Omega 6 fatty acid, found in many vegetable oils (e.g. sunflower oil). Alpha-linolenic acid is an essential Omega 3 fatty acid, present in many seed oils (e.g. chia, rapeseed, flaxseed, soy).
- An inappropriate ratio of Omega 6: Omega 3 can lead to numerous diseases, including cancer. Humans evolved to eat Omega 6: Omega 3 in a ratio of about 1:1, but today, many of us eat far too much Omega 6, distorting that ratio to about 10:1, and sometimes as high as 30:1.
- We must eat Omega 6: Omega 3 in the correct ratio. In other words, we should try and avoid sources of Omega 6 and eat more foods containing Omega 3 instead.
- A very important Omega 3 fatty acid is *docosahexaenoic acid* (DHA). It can be made in the body from alpha-linolenic acid or eaten in the diet. Oily fish (mackerel, tuna, sardines, salmon etc) is a good source of DHA.

Fats and inflammation

How do we react to a cut or a bruise? We get redness, pain, swelling and heat at the site of the wound, as our immune system gets to grips with the particular trauma in question.

We recognise this as inflammation, but a similar reaction takes place inside our bodies – out of sight and out of mind – whenever we stress our cells and tissues in some way. It seems that this internal inflammation not only leads to serious chronic diseases (heart disease, increased risk of cancer etc), but is directly related to obesity and the 'diseases of civilisation', including type 2 diabetes.[16]

So, what causes this inflammation? There are a number of possible reasons but pretty high on the list is – yes, you guessed it – modern, processed foods. One of the major culprits is sugar, but inflammation is also caused by an Omega 6 fatty acid called *arachidonic acid*; this particular Omega 6 fatty acid also raises the level of the hormone insulin, which as we will see later also causes untold problems. However, if we eat sufficient quantities of Omega 3 in our diet, we increase the level of another type of Omega 3 fatty acid called *DHA*, which has powerful anti-inflammatory effects. Unfortunately, most of us eat a diet that is way too high in Omega 6 fats and correspondingly too low in Omega 3 fats, which contributes to the internal inflammation that is so damaging to our health.

Re-establishing a healthy relationship with natural fat

The Back to Basics diet will help you re-establish a healthy relationship with fat by controlling your saturated fat intake and rebalancing your Omega 6: Omega 3 ratio by switching you over to a predominantly vegetarian diet. Now, before you throw this book in the bin in disgust, remember that this is not the same as eating an *exclusively* vegetarian diet. You will eat plenty of proteins, such as fish, chicken, turkey and the occasional piece of (organic) meat, but will just eat a lot more fruit, salad and vegetables along the way. Nevertheless, we can gain virtually all our daily fat needs by adding a small number of vegetarian foods to our diet. A good example is flaxseed, which you can buy in powdered form and just sprinkle over salads and vegetables. Flaxseed, otherwise known as linseed, has been around for thousands of years, but it is only recently that scientists have begun to realise just what a 'wonder food' flax might be. It is naturally low in carbohydrate and bursting with wonderful phytonutrients, but above all, it has high levels of Omega 3 fatty acids.

Other good sources of Omega 3 include walnuts, soy and tofu. I also heartily recommend a wonderful product called Udo's oil (www.udoerasmus.com), which I add to all my salads and many other meals. It has a lovely nutty flavour and has a perfect blend of organic oils, including Omega 9 (a non-essential fatty acid) in the correct ratio. Udo's oil is readily available nowadays in health food shops and online and is an excellent way to get your daily fats in the right amount and proportion. I must stress that I have no commercial relationship with this product or company – I simply genuinely like it and suggest you give it a go, too.

Trans fats – the real fat enemy!

Although I am convinced sugar is the real villain in our modern diet, the trans fats are a major cause of both the obesity epidemic and associated ill health seen today all around the World.[18,19] Sometimes referred to as *hydrogenated* fats, these are fats that are not natural in nature, but are instead manufactured by the food industry to extend the shelf life of processed foods. Natural polyunsaturated and monounsaturated fats are changed by '*hydrogen-ation*' (the artificial addition of hydrogen atoms to break the double bonds in the fatty acid chains, thereby creating a man-made saturated fat). This gives big profits to the food industry as such fats can resist oxidation (going rancid) for much longer than a natural fat. All in all, these fats are bad news. The Back to Basics diet has no place for these unnatural, man-made fats whatsoever, so wave trans fats a fond farewell and blow them a big kiss goodbye because you will not be seeing them again. Ever.

Our body fat is a warehouse, not an archive!

Unfortunately, our bodies work in the same way today as they did when humans first appeared on this Earth. This means our bodies still think we are living in the Stone Age; consequently, we lay down fat when food is plentiful for use on a rainy day. When food is scarce, as it was throughout much of human history, we are supposed to live off this fat reserve until such time we can again find something to eat. However,

WEIGHT LOSS THROUGH A VEGETARIAN DIET? NOT NECESSARILY.

- We are designed, by evolution, to eat a predominantly vegetarian diet.
- A *properly* constructed vegetarian diet might well be our healthiest diet.
- However, many vegetarians eat foods that are both unhealthy and fattening; a diet of cheese, pizza, bread, crisps, chips (French Fries) and sugary soft drinks is vegetarian but most definitely not a healthy, weight loss diet.
- By adding some natural (organic) meat, fish and fat to a predominantly vegetarian diet, we can put together a low-calorie, healthy way of eating that we can stick to for life (as per the Back to Basics diet in part two).
- Therefore, unless you are barred on religious, ethical or moral grounds, eating certain animals and fish is a sensible way to obtain the complete range of nutrients we need for a healthy diet.
- By all means become vegetarian if you wish; just remember that a vegetarian diet will need more care and attention in order to balance nutrients and calories than our natural diet, as recommended in part two.

most of us nowadays never use our fat reserves – we just add to them all of the time. Much of what follows in this book is a detailed explanation of how to switch over to burning fat so we lose weight, just as Nature intended. This is quite natural and in keeping with how we evolved to function as fit, healthy human beings. Our body fat is a warehouse, not an archive.

There is a lot of information here about fats, but it is a complicated subject that is often misunderstood. Come back to this section from time to time to refresh your memory, as an understanding of fats in particular is essential when we come to put together our new diet in part two. For now, though, let's leave fats alone and move on to look at our last class of *macronutrients*: the carbohydrates.

Carbohydrates

Carbohydrates or 'carbs' pretty much hold the key to our weight loss story. In one way or another, carbs dominate the diet industry – the 'high-carb, low-fat' diet, the 'low-carb' diet, the 'low-carb, high-fat' diet etc. I suspect you are as confused about all this as I was when I started researching this whole subject. I will let you into a secret; many of the 'low-carb' diets are on the right track, but very few of them seem to have grasped the whole story. In fact, everything about getting fat hinges on *processed* carbohydrates – the true villain of our story. Processed carbs are carbohydrates that have been changed in some way (e.g. wheat turned into flour into bread). In fact, I firmly believe that the root cause of the obesity epidemic is the availability of heavily processed, highly calorific carbohydrate foods everywhere we look! Carbs are obviously an important part of our story, so let's take a closer look at this rather infamous foodstuff.

Carbohydrates are made from sugar

Carbohydrates are the sugars and starch we all love to hate. Most carbs are built up from small molecules called *monosaccharides* (e.g. glucose, fructose and galactose). These used to be known as 'simple sugars' and form the building blocks of more complex carbohydrates. Monosaccharides can be linked together to form a *disaccharide* (e.g. sucrose or table sugar, which is made from glucose and fructose) and then on pretty much ad infinitum to something called a *polysaccharide*. Most carbohydrates are made by one of Nature's more amazing chemical processes: *photosynthesis*. Photosynthesis, fundamental to life on Earth, takes place in the green parts of plants. Here, light energy from the Sun is used to combine carbon dioxide from the atmosphere with water to make carbohydrate (glucose) and oxygen:

PHOTOSYNTHESIS (THE KEY TO LIFE ON EARTH)

(Light energy from the sun)
carbon dioxide + water = carbohydrate (glucose) + Oxygen

Much of the food we are designed to eat contains carbohydrate (e.g. fruits and vegetables). However, many of the foods we live on today are made from processed carbohydrate and as we shall see, it is these foods that cause us problems. Such processed carbohydrate foods include bread, pastries, pasta, white rice, sweets, soft drinks, beer, fried potatoes, cakes and chocolates. If you take nothing else from the book, please remember this key fact: carbohydrates are made from *sugar*. This includes foods that appear savoury to our taste (e.g. white bread, pasta, white rice).

Carbohydrates in their natural form are a vital part of the human diet, but things start to go wrong when we humans (aka the food industry) start messing around with carbohydrates in an attempt to mass-produce cheap, easily distributable food. Unfortunately, such processed carbs are everywhere and make up the bulk of many people's diets, often with disastrous consequences. [20,21]

By the way, there are no such things as essential carbohydrates. We can live perfectly happily as humans in a carbohydrate-free world. Don't worry – I am not going to advocate a carb-free diet.[22] We will talk about how carbs fit into our new, healthy diet at some length later in the book; for now, though, just remember that we don't actually need to eat carbs at all.

The problem of starch

Plants store energy in the form of starch, a polysaccharide made from lots of glucose linked together by chemical bonds. Starch is found in abundance in well-known foods such as potatoes and grains (e.g. wheat). When we eat starch, the large starch molecule is broken down to glucose by our digestive system, leading to lots of glucose molecules entering the blood stream. Glucose is an important fuel (and the main food for our brains), but the digestion of starch can be a double-edged sword, as *excess* glucose in the bloodstream will cause us problems – as we will later see.

Sugar – the root cause of our obesity

I hope you are starting to realise that excessive carbohydrate consumption might well be a bad thing because carbs are ultimately made of sugar? There is much confusion about all this, so let's just deal with the whole question of sugar now and try to understand why a high-sugar diet is just about the worst diet we could ever follow.[23]

When I first read the book *Eat to Live* by Dr Joel Fuhrman[24], I was struck by his explanation of how our health is governed by the ratio of calories to nutrients in our diet. I call this the 'Fuhrman Equation' as it is such a clever and succinct way of summing up how we should eat. In a nutshell, the 'Fuhrman Equation' is this:

$$\text{"Health} = \text{Nutrients/Calories}$$
$$\text{or, in algebraic terms, 'H'} = \text{N/C"}$$

In other words, our health is governed by the ratio of nutrients to calories in our diet, with the best health score derived from a diet that is very high in nutrients but correspondingly low in calories. Where does sugar fit into this scenario? Well, many experts describe sugar as an *anti-nutrient*, for the simple fact that sugar supplies excessive calories for essentially no nutritional benefit. Basically, sugar is a *non-nutrient*. Yes, sugar supplies calories, but it is not really a natural part of the human diet – early wild fruits were not terribly sweet. Some sugars can even be classed as toxins, much like alcohol and recreational drugs.

Sugar does many other nasty things to us as well. There is very good evidence that excess sugar consumption not only leads to obesity, but is a major contributory factor in type 2 diabetes and heart disease.[25] Even more disturbing is the suggestion that sugar is implicated in a number of cancers, including breast, colon and stomach cancer. There is startling new evidence suggesting how sugar consumption leads to all these various illnesses, as we will see later.

The two key dietary sugars are glucose and fructose (see box). Much of the reason we get so fat today is because of very high levels of these sugars (particularly fructose) in our modern diet.

It's time to 'let go' of sugar

Dietary processed sugar is so far away from what we should be eating, we need to leave it behind us now, once and for all. Let's just accept that sugar in all its forms (e.g. processed carbohydrate, soft drinks, beer, sweets, cakes, chocolates, table sugar etc) is something we ate in our previous life as overweight, unhealthy people. We need to wave all forms

SUGAR
(THE REASON WE ARE ALL FAT!)

- Sugar supplies excess calories for no nutritional benefit.
- Excess sugar consumption (mostly in the form of processed carbohydrate) is directly linked to obesity.
- Excess sugar consumption is a major contributing factor to type 2 diabetes.
- Sugar is implicated in a number of cancers, including breast, colon and stomach cancer.
- Sugar is very addictive – and the food industry knows this.
- To re-establish a healthy relationship with food and lose weight, unnecessary sugar (some fruit is fine) must be stripped from the diet.

of sugar a fond farewell and move on with our lives in a new, healthy direction. Nobody said this would be easy; sugar is one of the most addictive substances we could ever eat. However, if you want to change, I mean *really* change your life, you are going to have to make some tough decisions.

So just like quitting smoking, let's 'stub out' that dietary sugar. Stop, finished, gone. OK, happy now? You should be because you have changed something fundamental in your life that will allow you to regain control of your weight and long-term health. You are already well on the way to the new you. Well done!

So, which carbohydrates *should* we eat?

Most of us eat a diet that is packed full of carbohydrates. Many of our common foods (e.g. most breakfast cereals, bread, soft drinks, beer, pastry, potatoes, rice, pasta, sweets, chocolates, cakes etc) are all carbohydrates. What are carbohydrates made from? Sugar! So, in reality, many of us eat a diet that is almost exclusively made from sugar, which ends up as varying amounts of glucose and fructose in our bloodstream.

However, it is the rate at which a carbohydrate food ends up as glucose in the bloodstream that is crucial in determining our chances of putting on weight. In fact, most processed carbohydrates not only give us unnecessary calories, but also play havoc with our body chemistry in a way that makes it much more likely we will lay down fat, compared to the carbs contained in real, natural foods. Real, natural carbohydrate foods (e.g. fruits, salads, vegetables, a little brown rice, some quinoa, seeds, nuts etc) have none of the damaging effects of bad carbs, but will instead form the basis of a healthy, natural diet for the rest of your life. That's why the meal plans and dietary advice in part two will take care of your carbs for you, without you having to resort to charts or tables in the future.

The Glycaemic Index

Although natural carbohydrate foods should make up the bulk of our diet, most of us are overweight because our diet

GLUCOSE AND FRUCTOSE
(TWO KEY SUGARS)

- Glucose: glucose is made by plants during photosynthesis and is the end product of most carbohydrate digestion. Glucose is a perfectly natural human food source. Glucose is the fuel of choice for important organs such as the brain, kidneys and red blood cells. However, excess glucose in our bloodstream is a very bad thing and leads directly to obesity.

- Fructose: fructose is found in small quantities in fruit (and so can be considered a natural food), but most fructose is eaten as part of sucrose or table sugar. There has been a huge increase in fructose consumption since the 1960s (especially in the US), after corn began to be used to make High Fructose Corn Syrup or HFCS.

  Later, HFCS began to replace the more expensive cane sugar in foods such as sodas, burger buns, sweets and chocolates (today, these are available all around the World). Fructose is particularly dubious as unlike glucose, which has an important dietary role, it is treated by our metabolism much like alcohol – a known toxin. Just like alcohol, fructose is processed exclusively in the liver where it is converted to fat. Clearly, eating too much fructose is a bad thing to do.

contains far too many carbs. This apparent confusion is easily explained if we use something called the Glycaemic

Index (GI) to categorise the carbs in our diet. Many of you will have heard of this as it is referred to quite often in other diet literature.

Invented in the early 1980s, the GI ranks carbohydrate foods against a reference of glucose in terms of how quickly the carbohydrate food in question raises our blood sugar level.[26, 27] Glucose is given a value of one hundred on the Index, while the lowest point on the index is zero (i.e. no effect on blood sugar levels at all). Foods containing carbohydrates are ranked against glucose; the idea is that glucose is glucose, so obviously is top in terms of affecting the corresponding blood glucose concentration. Foods high on the index cause rapid increases in blood glucose levels, while foods low on the index show a much slower (or lesser) blood glucose response.

Most foods that are low on the index (which is good) are fruits, vegetables, some legumes and grains in their natural state. Most of the foods high on the index are processed carbohydrates (e.g. white bread, chips, cornflakes, ice cream, tomato ketchup etc). The GI is not perfect and there are other indices that are more useful in the real world (e.g. the Glyceamic Load index, which attempts to account for portion size as well and the 'Insulin Index', which ranks foods as to their effects on the secretion of insulin – the main topic in the next chapter). However, all this is largely academic, and the Back to Basics diet complies with all of these various indices quite naturally, without us having to refer back to them in the future.

That's the food science done. Hooray! Pat yourself on the back, as you are now well on the way to changing your life for the better forever. It is now time to lift the lid on certain aspects of our body chemistry that hold the key to understanding the real reasons why we get fat and why we find it so hard to lose weight on our modern diet.

So, let's roll up our sleeves and look in detail at the real culprits behind the causes of obesity: those remarkable chemical messengers we know as *hormones.*

Chapter 4 summary:

- Our modern diet is making us fat because it is completely out of kilter with our biological design.

- Proteins are an essential part of the human diet. Although we derive much of our protein from eating meat and fish, we can actually satisfy all our protein needs with a balanced vegetarian diet.

- Fats have had a very bad press. In fact, however, fats are an essential part of the natural human diet.

- Processed carbohydrate lies at the heart of the current obesity epidemic. However, carbohydrates in real food should make up the bulk of our diet.

5

Lose weight and stay young forever?
Your hormones hold the key!

In this important chapter, you will see why:

- Numerous hormones are intimately involved in controlling our appetite and deciding whether or not we gain weight.

- Most of us are no longer sensitive to the appetite control hormone known as leptin – one of our natural calorie counters.

- The role and function of the hormone insulin is central to the causes of obesity.

- High levels of insulin, caused primarily by the overconsumption of processed carbohydrate, leads directly to weight gain.

- Low levels of insulin in the bloodstream decrease the use of glucose and promote 'fat burning', so we lose weight.

- Low levels of insulin might, just might, hold the key to eternal youth, too.

The story so far

We have looked at the make-up and content of the foods we eat today and have discussed why these types of food differ from the foods we are designed, by evolution, to eat. We have also seen that our modern diet, full of processed carbohydrate, trans fats, sugars and excess calories, somehow leads to inexorable weight gain. And we are constantly being told to 'eat less and move more' because calories ultimately dictate our weight. Or do they…?

Our body chemistry is identical to that of our Stone Age ancestors.

We digest and process our food in exactly the same way as our ancestors. In other words, our body chemistry, identical to that of our hunter-gatherer predecessors, has evolved over eons of time under what we can call the original human diet.[1] This is the diet everyone ate, for hundreds and thousands of years, before we 'ruined' everything by inventing agriculture. The original human diet contained real, natural foods, which were relatively low in calories (compared to the types of foods most of us eat today) but high in nutrients. Here is a reminder of a typical ancestral diet:

- High levels of naturally occurring plant material.

- Reasonable amounts of animal protein and fat.

- Very low levels of sugar (compared to our diet today).

- Absolutely no processed food.

- Relatively low amounts of calories (compared to our diet today).

This type of diet, when combined with plenty of daily exercise, kept our ancestors fit and healthy and gave them enough calories for their hard, demanding lives. During the summer months or after a successful hunt, they would have been able to lay down some fat reserves to see them through the hard times when food was scarce. However, as far as we can tell, they were not obese; in fact, they would have spent most of their lives perpetually hungry, frantically searching for their next meal.[2]

To survive, they would have had to access and live off their fat reserves to keep them going until such time they could hunt or gather their next meal. So, part of our ancestral legacy is a fat double-edged sword – we are very efficient at storing fat (so we put on weight), but also have the means to use that fat for fuel (so we lose weight) when food is scarce. Today, most of us are experts at the former and not so adept at the latter.

There is more to this story than calories

Obesity is a disease of excess calorie consumption, but that is only part of the story. Most of us do eat too many calories, largely because modern foods contain unnaturally high levels of calories and we eat these foods far too often.[3] This probably explains why we are so adept at storing fat because we are eating far more calories than our ancestors ever did. However, this doesn't explain why we then struggle to lose weight by using our fat reserves for fuel or why modern foods seem to make us so fat so easily, or why many of us develop type 2 diabetes and other 'diseases of civilisation' as our weight spirals out of control?

To understand why our modern diet is so destructive to both our health and our waistline, we need to look beyond the simplistic 'calories in – calories out' idea and the 'eat less, move more' mantra to find the real reasons behind our galloping obesity. The answer lies in the remarkable interplay of certain hormones that ultimately control both our appetite and how we manage the fat stores around our body.[4, 5] Our modern diet upsets these hormones to such an extent that we develop various chronic conditions, including obesity.

Our hormones hold the key to weight loss

Many of you will have heard of hormones and probably regard them with disdain – puberty, acne, menstruation, the menopause, obesity, sexual drive (or otherwise), growth and

HORMONES

- Hormones are *proteins* that are made in glands of the *endocrine system* (e.g. the pituitary, thyroid, adrenal glands, pancreas etc), before being secreted into the bloodstream to do their work somewhere else.
- Hormones control numerous processes in our bodies (e.g. puberty, acne, menstruation, the menopause etc).
- Hormones are *directly* involved in our obesity.
- The foods we eat in our modern diet (particularly processed carbohydrate) disturbs certain hormones systems (e.g. insulin and leptin), resulting in weight gain.
- Although the calories in our diet ultimately decide whether or not we put on weight, if our food hormones are disturbed by our modern diet, it is very hard to avoid putting on weight (or subsequently to lose weight), however hard we try.

changes during pregnancy are all affected by hormones. Hormones are just chemical messengers that are usually made in one part of the body, but tell a system elsewhere to do a particular job.

By looking at how certain hormones work in and around the digestion of our food, we can begin to piece together the story of why we get so fat so easily on our modern diet. What we find is that processed foods and sugar disturb these hormones in such a way that it is almost impossible to avoid putting on weight. [6,7]

Our food hormones

If you look up on the Internet the reasons why people gain weight, you will unearth a whole list of hormones that are intimately involved in various aspects of obesity. Any number of these plays an important role in the technical aspect of weight gain (e.g. *ghrelin*, a hormone secreted in the stomach that stimulates our appetite). In fact, one of the benefits of *bariatric* (weight loss) surgery seems to be the removal of ghrelin-producing cells when large chunks of the stomach are cut out. Many other chemicals and hormones (e.g. peptide YY) are also crucial in stimulating or blunting our appetites. However, I have decided here to concentrate on just two primary 'food' hormones, because I believe they are the most important in the whole obesity story.

One of these hormones is *insulin* which, in combination with excess calorie consumption, I consider to be the main factor in all things to do with obesity.[8, 9] We'll discuss insulin in a moment, but first of all, I want to talk about *leptin* – a hormone involved in controlling our appetite and hence one that is often the cause of us having eyes bigger than our stomachs!

Leptin – our appetite hormone

Leptin is a hormone secreted from our own fat cells and is designed to tell us that our fat reserves are full, so stop eating! Leptin levels are directly proportional to levels of *adipose* tissue. In English, this means that the fatter the person, the more leptin they produce. How can this be? Surely more leptin should signal less eating? Yes, that's true, but something has obviously gone wrong with our ability to respond to leptin, otherwise no one would be overweight or fat.

If we consider obesity from an evolutionary perspective, excess eating is costly and just plain unnecessary. It would have been much easier for a Stone Age man or woman to survive the winter by putting on about 10 stone of fat; however, such obesity would have made it impossible for them to run away from predators or otherwise be a useful member of the tribe. In the natural world, there is no such thing as a free lunch; so, evolution came up with leptin. Once sufficient fat reserves had been laid down, leptin would signal "I'm full" and life would continue without having to eat all the time. So, what has gone so wrong today? Unfortunately, it is all down to our modern high-sugar diet (more on leptin later).

Insulin – the master hormone

Insulin is the key to determining whether you or I will be a slim person or a fat person during our lifetime. We mustn't lose sight of the fact that, ultimately, calories determine our weight, but if we can understand how insulin works in an around the digestion of our food, we will be well on our way to banishing our obesity forever.

It is a pretty sure bet that those of us who are overweight have a dysfunctional insulin mechanism (i.e. we are resistant to the message insulin is trying to send.[12, 13]) How we respond to insulin underpins everything we need to know about obesity, but the actual cause of this 'insulin resistance' is still not completely understood. It seems either something in our modern diet upsets the normal mechanism of insulin, so that far too much insulin is produced far too often, or our obesity – caused through excess calorie consumption – has stopped us recognising insulin's message. Either way, the important point is that we are no longer responding to insulin the way we should.

Some research scientists argue that all that matters in obesity is calories; others feel that any one of a whole suite of other body systems might be involved in making us fat. Nevertheless, the concept of insulin resistance is pretty much central to any theory about why our modern diet makes us fat. Tackling insulin resistance is therefore a key part of the Back to Basics diet; it is only by managing our calories *and* our insulin levels that we can rid ourselves of our obesity, once and for all.

So, what does insulin do?

Insulin's main role is to work in conjunction with another hormone to balance our blood sugar levels. Blood sugar? What has this got to do with putting on weight? Well, this may surprise you, but this blood sugar system – so badly messed up by our modern diet – is also central to our body's control of our weight.

Pretend for a moment we have been transported back in time to the Stone Age (or the *Paleolithic* Era, to be more scientific) where, through the miracle of our imagination, we can look in on a typical couple sitting down to a meal in the comfort of their cave. They are about to eat real, unprocessed foods – the foods that fed our ancestors for hundreds and thousands of years. Remember that our body chemistry developed over that huge span of time under this very same sort of diet. What were these real foods? Mostly plant foods, some meat and fish, eggs, nuts, seeds and natural fats. So, let's look at how these foods, the foods we are *designed* to eat, affect our blood sugar levels.

Why our blood sugar levels are so important

Many of our cells, tissues and organs are fussy about what they eat. Our brains, in particular, rely almost exclusively on a regular supply of *glucose* in the blood, often referred to as blood sugar. If we were stranded on a desert island, starving, our bodies could make an alternative 'brain food' called a *ketone* by breaking down our own muscles. Fortunately, under normal conditions, the preferred food supply for the brain is glucose. However, our brains are *so* fussy about the amount of glucose they need that our blood sugar levels have to be maintained in an extremely narrow range of concentrations at all times or we are in trouble (Fig 5).

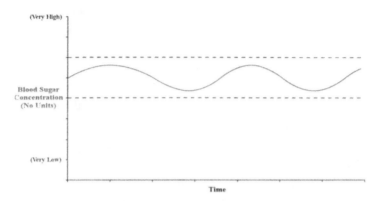

Fig 5. Blood sugar levels are maintained in a narrow range of concentrations at all times.

What is this ideal concentration of blood sugar? Well, imagine a 5-litre bucket of water stood on a table – if I stir in just one teaspoon of table sugar into the 5 litres of water (roughly equivalent to the total blood volume of an average person), that's about the concentration of blood sugar that we have to maintain all the time to keep our brains happy. Just a bit more sugar is toxic, while a slightly lower concentration also causes us problems, too. Remember, we are talking about the equivalent of one teaspoon of sugar, give or take a little bit.

The ancestral diet, the diet we are designed to eat, allows our hormones to balance our blood sugar levels easily and efficiently, just as Nature intended. However, our high-sugar modern diet puts this blood sugar system under enormous pressure, which, as we'll see, leads directly to obesity.[16]

An ancestral diet allows our hormones to balance our blood sugar

Let's return to our *Paleo* couple, now happily lying about in their cave digesting their dinner of antelope meat and greens – fine dining in those days! This sort of food takes quite a long time to digest – unprocessed plant food, in particular, is difficult to break down. Consequently, the *glucose* from the plant food, plus the amino acids from proteins, is drip-fed into the bloodstream in the hours following their meal. Let's now zoom in and look at how the digestion of this type of natural food, in particular the digestion of carbohydrate, affects the hormones inside our bodies that are trying to manage our blood sugar levels. Remember, these hormones affect whether or not we gain or lose weight.

Insulin gets to work

As the glucose, amino acids and fatty acids pass into the bloodstream of our *Paleo* couple, their blood sugar concentration slowly starts to rise. This will happen to you and me as well, if we eat in the same way. This is all perfectly normal, but we know this rise in blood sugar has to be controlled or we will damage our brains. In fact, if your blood sugar levels get too high, a doctor will tell you that you have *hyperglycaemia* (US: *hyperglycemia*) or too much sugar in the blood (Fig 6). So, somehow we have to juggle using glucose as a fuel source for our cells and tissues, but keep the concentration of glucose in the blood at safe levels.

To get around this problem, the amazing power of evolution and natural selection has come up with the hormone *insulin* as a way of managing our blood sugar levels. This is one part of a relatively simple but exquisitely controlled feedback system controlled through the pancreas.

Our much-abused pancreas

After a meal, clever biochemical sensing systems in the pancreas notice the rising levels of glucose in the blood. In response, cells in one part of the pancreas (beta cells) secrete *insulin* into the bloodstream. In the case of our *Paleo* couple, only a small

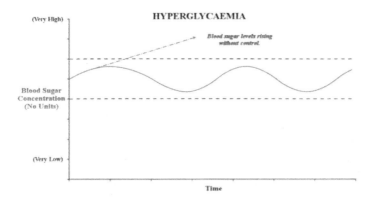

Fig 6. If blood sugar levels rise too much, we risk a dangerous condition known as 'hyperglycaemia'.

amount of insulin will be needed because glucose is only drip-fed into the bloodstream for some time after their meal of antelope and sides. This sort of food results in a relatively slow rise in blood sugar levels. And because this type of real food does *not* cause a rapid spike in blood sugar concentration, the corresponding insulin response is minimal, too.

OK, but what exactly does insulin do? Insulin has many functions, but in terms of our body weight, insulin rebalances our blood sugar levels by *removing excess glucose* from the bloodstream.[17] In the case of our *Paleo* couple, we know that only a small amount of insulin is required to smooth out their mildly elevated blood sugar levels. Once this has been achieved, levels of insulin in the bloodstream return to a 'ticking over' background level, in preparation for performing exactly the same role at the next meal (Fig 7).

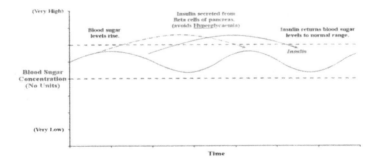

Fig 7. How insulin returns blood sugar levels to normal, so avoiding hyperglycaemia.

So, insulin has done its job by helping our *Paleo* couple avoid hyperglycaemia. They can now use the glucose from their meal for energy to power them through their undoubtedly hard lives. If we follow this type of original human diet ourselves, we can also fill up on low-calorie, highly nutritious plant food, which then takes a long time to digest. This allows glucose to be drip-fed into *our* bloodstream, so that we can easily manage blood sugar levels. This is how our bodies are designed to work.

Too much insulin makes us fat

Insulin levels will rise even if we just eat protein, but most insulin is secreted in response to eating sugar. The more sugar you eat, the more insulin your pancreas has to produce. However, we know our blood sugar levels have to be kept at the equivalent of one teaspoon of sugar in our entire blood volume. So, where does this excess glucose go? Some of it will be used immediately for fuel by various cells and tissues (e.g. in the muscles of very active people such as our Paleo ancestors or modern-day endurance athletes). However, any remaining glucose is stored in the body as a reserve of energy, available later in times of fasting. This is insulin's key role – excess glucose is swept out of the bloodstream and stored for a rainy day. [18]

So, we know that insulin, an energy storage or *anabolic* hormone, keeps blood sugar concentrations at the correct level by removing excess glucose from the bloodstream. So the next question is, how and where is all this excess glucose stored? Well, first of all, it is stored in the liver and muscles in the form of *glycogen*, a short-term energy source available for immediate use. However, once glycogen stores are full, any remaining glucose is stored as fat.

Insulin drives excess blood sugar to fat

How does insulin turn blood sugar into glycogen and fat? Well, it all begins when an insulin molecule binds to the surface of a cell in the liver – a biochemical version of the space shuttle docking with the space station. Through the magic of biochemistry, this 'docking' of the insulin molecule to cell wall creates an opening into the cell. Excess glucose molecules in the bloodstream are then ushered in through this opening, where they are converted in the cell to glycogen. This same process also takes place in muscle cells – another region of glycogen storage. Glycogen is evolution's answer to the sabre-toothed tiger; when you need to run away from something with big teeth fast, you use your glycogen reserve for immediate energy.

Most humans can store about 400 grams of glycogen in total, which provides less than two hours' worth of energy during strenuous exercise. Our *Paleo* couple, active all day long, would have used their glycogen stores a lot and so would have replenished their glycogen stores at every meal. Unfortunately, for those of us today who are sedentary, our glycogen reserves are pretty much full all the time.

When glycogen stores are full, the body faces a quandary. Blood sugar levels still need to be controlled, so what happens now to any remaining excess glucose in the blood? Under the influence of insulin, any remaining glucose and *triglycerides* in the bloodstream are now stored as fat in our fat cells or *adipose* tissue. The higher the levels of insulin, the more of this storage occurs. Yes, too much fat in our diet will make things worse (independent of insulin, actually), but it is largely a myth that eating too much fat makes you fat. The main cause of obesity is the overconsumption of sugar and processed carbs, mediated through our poor old, used and abused insulin system.

So, pause for effect. Write this on the back of your hand, across your computer screen or tattoo it on your forehead (only joking), but please remember that:

- Carbohydrates are made from sugar. Excess (processed) carbohydrate consumption leads to elevated blood sugar levels (*hyperglycaemia*), which in turn leads to elevated levels of insulin, which ultimately makes us gain weight.

Maintaining low insulin levels is the key to weight loss

Most of us eat in a way that keeps our insulin levels high, all day long. Evolution has designed us to survive periods of famine by relying on the fat reserves around our body. This means that when we are truly hungry, we need some sort of mechanism to 'open the warehouse door' of our fat reserves so that we can live off our fat for a while, at least until our next meal. Unfortunately, this is the side of our fat metabolism that we are not very good at today.

Imagine we have long since finished digesting our last meal, our stomachs are empty and we are getting hungry. Insulin levels will now be low because we are not consuming food – there is no need for high levels of insulin in the bloodstream at this point. Actually, insulin starts to be secreted when we anticipate food, such as when we walk into the kitchen and smell that lovely roast dinner in the oven. And guess what, when insulin levels are low, fat burning (through a process called *lipolysis*) is stimulated. This is evolution's answer to living in a world where food supply was decidedly intermittent; when insulin levels are low, we are able to breakdown our body fat for use as fuel to power our lives – exactly how we are designed to work.

Now, here's the kicker. *High* levels of insulin in the blood *inhibit* lipolysis, meaning our bodies are unable to burn fat.[19] It was previously thought that another hormone (glucagon – more in a moment) stimulated lipolysis, but recent research indicates that it is more to do with low levels of insulin kick-starting the fat-burning process.[20] The details, as always, are complicated, but the key point is this: if we spend our lives permanently insulinated (i.e. with high levels of insulin in our bloodstream), it is very hard to lose weight regardless of calorie consumption. To burn fat away from around our bodies and regain control of our own health destiny, we need to keep our insulin levels low as much as possible.

What happens if we don't eat for a while?

How did our *Paleo* ancestors survive the hard times? Would they have starved to death had they not been able to find anything to eat for a day or two? No, they managed just fine because evolution has got this way of life covered – otherwise you and I would never have made it as the most successful species on the planet.

During periods of famine, our *Paleo* couple would have relied on their low insulin levels to help them access their body fat via the fat burning process known as lipolysis. However, by not eating for a while, is there not a danger that their blood sugar levels will fall too low? Yes, that is a distinct possibility, but we know that evolution has an answer for this as well. When blood sugar levels start to drop, a different hormone is secreted from the pancreas called *glucagon*. Through another remarkable series of actions, glucagon provides glucose for use as fuel from storage, while simultaneously rebalancing the concentration of glucose in the blood to the correct level. This stops our blood sugar level falling too low between meals – a condition known as *hypoglycaemia* or 'too little' glucose in the blood.

Insulin and glucagon control our blood sugar levels

So, between them, insulin and glucagon work in harmony to control our blood sugar levels (Fig 8). This is called a feedback system because as each hormone starts to exert its effect, the corresponding change in blood sugar levels is sensed once more in the pancreas and so less and less of the hormone is produced as a result. This means that under normal circumstances, such as our healthy *Paleo* couple, we are extremely sensitive to these two hormonal signals. Together, insulin and glucagon are more than capable of keeping our blood sugar at the correct level.[21]

In fact, glucagon can keep our blood sugar topped up for about three days before we need to eat anything at all. Insulin and glucagon are designed to work as a fine-tuning mechanism, ticking away in the background and balancing our blood sugar levels after infrequent, low-sugar meals. Insulin should be at a background or *basal* level for most of the day, only being secreted from the pancreas in very small quantities during and shortly after infrequent meals of unprocessed food. Evolution has designed us to live in a state of low insulin for most of the time[22].

The relationship between insulin and glucagon is fairly fixed and inflexible, much like a child's seesaw in a playground (Fig 9). In other words, we can't have high levels of insulin in the blood and high levels of glucagon at the same time. Insulin is produced in response to a meal and in particular, in response to carbohydrate (sugar) consumption. Conversely, glucagon is secreted in response to low blood sugar, normally some hours after a meal when insulin is necessarily at a low level.

OK, but what has all this got to do with losing weight? To lose weight we have to eat fewer calories than we burn

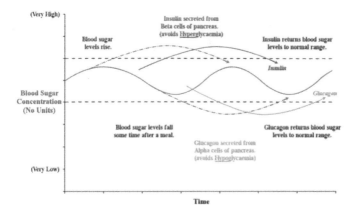

Fig 8. Insulin and glucagon combine in a feedback system to control blood sugar concentration at all times.

up. However, to really burn off that body fat once and for all, we have to spend as much time as possible in a state of low insulin. This way, we can start to live in accordance with our evolutionary design – we are not meant to eat sugary, fatty, processed carbohydrate foods all day long.

Consequently, on the Back to Basics diet, you will eat in a way that gives your poor pancreas a rest. You will not eat all the time, so your insulin levels will be able to drop back to idle as much as possible. Instead, you will enjoy plentiful, healthy, nutritious meals that will banish your obesity forever and allow you to regain control of your long-term health at the same time. Insulin is a vital hormone, but our modern diet plays havoc with our insulin mechanism such that our body is always trying to store our food energy for that famous rainy day. By managing our diet and lifestyle in a way that does not antagonise our insulin levels, we can put the final 'nail in the coffin' of our obesity once and for all.

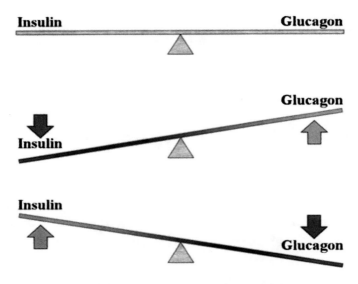

Fig 9. The interplay between insulin and glucagon.

The Back to Basics Diet and Insulin

On the Back to Basics programme, you will lose weight by eating fewer calories than you burn through the combination of a delicious, healthy, natural, real food diet and daily exercise (which we will refer to as activity.) You will also spend far more hours of the day in a state of low insulin, when lipolysis is activated, than in high insulin, where fat burning is severely impaired.

So, from now on, don't fret too much about the types of food on your plate – provided they are not processed foods. I am convinced that the best way to approach healthy weight loss is to eat a diet of predominantly vegetarian foods to reduce calorie consumption and boost nutrient intake, while minimising insulin levels at the same time. This type of food contains little sugar and is digested slowly; both these factors help to minimise insulin production.

If we then try and cut down the number of meals we eat to, for example, two a day and add in daily activity, we really put the mockers on insulin and give ourselves the best chance of changing the bad habits of a lifetime. By adopting a sensible, healthy way of eating, combined with daily activity, we can lose weight safely and easily and boost our health and happiness at the same time.

Stay young forever – another reason to control insulin?

I hope I have convinced you of the benefits of keeping your insulin levels low as much as possible. Nevertheless, exciting new science from America might make a low insulin lifestyle even more enticing.

We all get old, don't we? It's just one of those things. In fact, ageing has always been thought of as just a natural part

MANAGING OUR INSULIN
(The Victorian signal box)

- Imagine an old-fashioned signal box on the side of a railway line, full of huge levers that switch the points over. A Victorian gentleman, complete with waistcoat, peaked cap and bushy moustache, is grasping one of those levers on our behalf.

- You have just woken up – glucagon levels are high, insulin levels are low (we don't need insulin when we are asleep – there isn't any excess glucose overnight because we are fasting). We are now primed for weight loss. In other words, if we don't eat anything for a few hours, our energy needs would have to be met through fat burning, mediated by our low insulin levels, rather than from food.

- Imagine instead that we have just tumbled out of bed, put on the kettle and grabbed a bowl of cereal and a couple of rounds of white toast with butter and marmalade (sound familiar?). What happens in the signal box now? The signalman will switch our body chemistry from a 'fasting' state (with glucagon in the ascendancy) to a 'fed' state (where insulin is secreted in response to food, especially if we eat a high-carbohydrate meal).

- In the 'fed' state, our body wants to store food energy. Consequently, it is very hard to lose weight in the 'fed' state. We have to wait for a few hours after a meal for insulin to return to a background level, which will again stimulate lipolysis so we can use our 'warehouse' of fat for fuel once again.

of life. However, two recently discovered genes (in a worm!) might hold the key to a dramatically longer life for all of us, free from disease and all the normal signs of ageing, including getting fat. [23, 24]

Genes are sections of our DNA that contain a code of some sort, which when turned on tell our body to 'do' or 'make' something. Remarkably, it seems that if we change what we eat (yes, back to real food and away from insulin-spiking processed carbs and sugar), we might be able to control these particular genes so that we can delay ageing and avoid many of the normal symptoms of old age. OK, these genes were found in worms, but it seems likely they exist in humans as well.

The scientist who discovered these genes nicknamed the first one the "Grim Reaper" because it seemed to code for all the normal signs of ageing. However, the second gene, which was nicknamed "Sweet Sixteen", had an amazing ability to confer youth in its host. It seems that an active "Grim Reaper" gene stops the youthful "Sweet Sixteen" gene from working, so ageing happens as per normal. Here is the startling fact, though – the "Grim Reaper" gene codes for a protein that allows certain cells and tissues to recognise a particular hormone. Can you guess what that hormone might be? An insulin-like hormone with an identical molecular shape to insulin! [25]

So, what does all this mean to us? Although there is a long way to go with the science yet, it does seem highly likely that these two genes exist in humans. So, if we can somehow switch off or at least restrict the action of the "Grim Reaper" gene by making less insulin, the "Sweet Sixteen" gene can start to work. This will lead to a remarkable cascade of good chemical reactions throughout the body, which to all intents and purposes keeps us young.

However, if we eat in a way that keeps the "Grim Reaper" gene switched on, the "Sweet Sixteen" gene will be turned off. We will then age and get fat as per normal, and risk all those nasty diseases we have already discussed. So, by eating so that we minimize our insulin response, we might be able to stave off old age – at least for a while. One day, no doubt, we'll be able to take a pill, which will let us live to one hundred with the body of a 30-year-old. In the meantime, this seems like another very good reason to adopt a low insulin lifestyle to me.

Chapter 5 summary:

- Leptin controls our appetite, while insulin and glucagon manage our blood sugar levels. Insulin sweeps excess glucose from the bloodstream and stores it as a reserve of energy, initially as glycogen. When glycogen stores are full, insulin enables the long-term storage of excess blood glucose as fat.

- If we eat too much sugar (or processed carbohydrate), we will raise our blood sugar levels too much, leading to high levels of insulin in the blood.

- High levels of insulin in the blood leads directly to weight gain; by contrast, low levels of insulin in the bloodstream decrease the use of glucose and instead promote lipolysis (i.e. fat burning), so we lose weight.

- On the Back to Basics diet, you will eat real foods that have a minimal effect on insulin levels. Add a little intermittent fasting with daily activity and we can break the habit of grazing all day long on processed foods. By remaining in a low insulin state most of the time, we can access our 'warehouse' of fat to fuel our daily lives.

- We might also (just might) live much longer without succumbing to the degenerative diseases of old age.

6

Fat? Our modern diet and lifestyle is to blame!

In this chapter, you will see why:

- Many of us are intolerant to the processed carbohydrates in our modern diet.

- Real plant foods are actually low-carb, contrary to popular belief.

- Our modern, high-sugar diet leads directly to internal inflammation, leading to insulin and leptin resistance and obesity.

- Insulin resistance is at the heart of the obesity epidemic. To lose weight effectively, we simply must eat in a way that returns us to insulin sensitivity.

- Too much insulin in the bloodstream can lead to type 2 diabetes.

- Resistance to leptin means we lose control of our appetite and eat too much.

- We don't need to eat all of the time – our hormones are perfectly capable of managing our blood sugar levels on a real food diet.

- The Back to Basics diet will reduce your calorie consumption and return you to hormonal sensitivity.

What have we learned so far?

Let's just pause for a moment and reflect on what we have learned so far. First of all, we have seen that being obese, overweight, 'tubby' – whatever you want to call it – is most definitely not our fault. We do have to accept that most of us today eat too many calories; however, this is mostly due to a complex web of circumstances involving a move away from our historical natural, real food diet and lifestyle to a modern way of life that is largely sedentary and involves eating far too much processed food. Combine this with hormones sent haywire by the contents of our food, resulting in a constant desire to eat (leptin) and a permanent state of fat deposition (insulin), is it any wonder we are all in such a mess with our weight?

Before we finally finish off all this part one science 'stuff', I want to touch on some other key aspects of a healthy diet that are often misunderstood or misinterpreted. I want to start by returning to the thorny subject of carbs. We have touched on the subject of carbs already, but as this whole aspect of diet and weight loss is such a minefield, I thought it would be useful to tidy up the 'carbohydrate story' once and for all before moving onto the diet plans themselves in part two. As we are about to see, a high-carbohydrate diet, one that seems to go against the grain (pardon the pun) of our new approach to food, might actually be the healthiest diet we could ever eat.

Carbs – friend *and* foe?

One of the most puzzling aspects of human nutrition is why certain populations (e.g. various traditional peoples who cling onto a hunter-gatherer lifestyle) seem to be in perfect health on diets containing very different types of macronutrient.

For instance, the Masai of East Africa traditionally live almost exclusively on a diet of milk, meat and blood, yet they are extremely lean and seem to be virtually free from any form of heart disease.[1] Similarly, the Turkana people of Kenya consume a predominantly meat-based diet, but avoid any signs of metabolic syndrome or other signs of ill health.[2] There are many other examples – including the Inuit and the native American Plains Indians of the 19th Century – of hunter-gatherer societies who have existed quite happily for generations on a diet of just meat and fat, while maintaining perfect health. However, numerous other non–Western groups, including the much-studied Kitavans of Papua New Guinea[3], live on a diet that is almost exclusively carbohydrate, while also remaining remarkably healthy.

How can this be? We know that too many carbs is a bad thing, so how can a high-carbohydrate diet be healthy? All these people take fairly high levels of daily activity, so are we just back to 'calories in – calories out' once again? Not necessarily – virtually all these disparate groups will get fat and succumb to the 'diseases of civilisation', if and when they are exposed to our Western diet.[4] In fact, non-Western people appear to suffer much more in terms of sudden onset obesity or type 2 diabetes etc when exposed to a Western diet, compared to those of European origin who have been exposed to the Western diet since birth[5,6]. So, the key seems to be that something in our diet is upsetting both our bodies and those of non-Western people when they abandon their traditional way of eating.

Carbohydrate intolerance

So far, we have 'pointed the finger' at carbohydrate as one of the main causes of obesity. For instance, we know that processed carbohydrates (sugar) play havoc with our insulin/glucagon system, leading directly to weight gain. However, this is just one example of the numerous damaging effects of our modern diet. In reality, most of us are basically allergic to these modern, processed foods, such that we find it very difficult to digest these foods without making ourselves ill and/or fat.

The term *carbohydrate intolerance* (CI) has been coined to explain our inability to properly digest the high-sugar foods of our modern diet.[7] Even if you do not currently have 'CI' and remain slim on a diet of processed carbohydrate foods, it is almost certain that you are storing up trouble for the future and will, in time, become ill like the rest of us. So, I quite understand why many nutritionists and diet authors promote a low-carb diet – put simply, if carbs make us ill (and obese), it makes sense to remove them from our diet. In terms of processed carbohydrate and other sources of sugar, I entirely agree. However, the danger is that *all* carbohydrates become tarred with the same brush, which, as we are about to see, is a serious mistake.

The Kitavans – the healthiest people on Earth?

The Kitavans live in Papua New Guinea and are reckoned to be one of the healthiest peoples on Earth. Most of their food consists of unprocessed carbohydrate (i.e. fruit and vegetables, especially root vegetables, together with limited amounts of meat and fish). What is obvious about these remarkable people is that they have no exposure whatsoever to modern, processed food – no grains or flour, no sugar and no nasty man-made oils or fats. In summary, the Kitavans, much like the Masai, the Turkana and most of the other Aboriginal peoples around the world, eat only natural and unprocessed food.

How can these people exhibit such astonishing health on a diet that is high in carbohydrate, when we believe that too much carbohydrate in the diet is a very bad thing? The answer is complex, but it all hinges on something known as *carbohydrate density*[8]. To understand this, we need to use our imagination again.

The low-carbohydrate density of real plant food

How do you think you would feel if, on Christmas morning, you gave your partner a very expensive box of chocolates, only to find that the box contained mostly tissue paper and packaging and only four individual chocolates? You would be cross, I suspect, but how would you describe the density of the chocolates in the box? Perhaps, you might say, they were *low* density.

Now, imagine that somebody has given you six of these chocolate boxes on Christmas morning? Lucky you! As an experiment, you open each box in turn, discard the tissue paper, tip each tray of chocolates into a bowl and throw away the tray. At the end of all of this, you have the chocolates from all six boxes in the bowl. You throw away all of the packaging but keep just one, now empty, box behind. Into this empty box, you tip all of the chocolates and replace the lid with satisfaction. Now how would you describe the density of chocolates in the one remaining box? It would be a very *high* density of chocolates now.

What has this got to do with carbohydrate? Plants store carbohydrate in their cells as starch, but the density of carbohydrate stored in unprocessed plant food (e.g. fruits, tubers, leaves etc) is really rather low, with a maximum density of about 23% by mass (the remaining 77% is mostly water). This is the equivalent density of our original box of chocolates.

By comparison, the processed carbohydrate we eat as the bulk of our modern diet is the equivalent of all the chocolates tipped into one box on Christmas morning! Consider wheat for a moment – we know that the food industry takes the seeds (grain) from wheat and subjects them to intensive processing in order to produce flour on an enormous scale. The milling process disrupts the cell walls of the wheat seed, which leads to the carbohydrate in each cell being released and concentrated into a sort of supercharged high-density carbohydrate (and high-calorie) product called flour. As we know, this is then turned into lots of naughty foods (bread, cakes, pasta etc).

Interestingly, carbohydrate density does not change during the cooking of real food, as the carbohydrate stays trapped inside the cell with only the joints between the cells themselves broken during the cooking process.

The Kitavans, in fact, eat a low-calorie, low-carb diet

Let's now return to the Kitavans and their carbohydrates. We know the Kitavans and those of us following a similar dietary regime eat only real plant foods and have no exposure to grains, flour and sugar. If we keep the idea of density from the above example in mind, the explanation for this apparent anomaly in carbohydrate consumption unfolds before our very eyes.

What is carbohydrate? Ultimately, it is sugar. Therefore, if we look closely at the diet of the Kitavans or others who appear to eat a high-carbohydrate diet with impunity, we find in fact that they are eating natural, real plant foods that have a low-carbohydrate density. This means the sugar content of such foods is similarly low, so they only experience a low insulin response on this type of diet. The Kitavans actually consume relatively few calories and have a limited insulin response to their diet. They are active all day long and have remarkably low levels of disease markers that are unfortunately all too common in many obese Western people. Such a diet naturally results in low levels of obesity, too. Eating a high-carb diet suddenly doesn't sound too bad, does it? Why, then, should our typical high-sugar Western diet, based on processed grains, added sugar and bad fats, be so damaging to our health? The answer is startling and not at all obvious – in fact, it probably comes down to the millions of bacteria living in our gut.

Our gut bacteria ultimately controls our weight

You may have heard of 'good' gut bacteria and the use of probiotics to encourage their growth? Once thought of as mostly 'out of sight and out of mind', such helpful bacteria now appears vital to our overall health and seems able to relieve many of the unpleasant symptoms of our modern diet, such as IBS. However, the balance of bacteria in our guts, often disturbed by our modern diet, might be a key factor in deciding whether or not we will gain weight[9, 10].

Many bacteria are classed as *Gram Negative* and have something called *bacterial lipopolysaccharide* (LPS) in their cell walls. Remarkably, it seems that high levels of LPS from 'bad' bacteria may actually lead directly to obesity. We humans, including the bacterial passengers inside our guts, evolved over millions of years under a dietary regime of real, unprocessed foods and virtually no sugar. This lack of sugar in the ancestral diet favoured a particular type of 'good' gut bacteria, which are helpful to us and form an important part of our digestive and immune systems.

However, our modern, high-sugar diet now favours different forms of bacteria that otherwise would not have much of a chance of establishing a foothold in our guts if we had continued to eat the food we are supposed to eat. Instead, these 'bad' bacteria now flourish and in evolutionary terms, they 'out compete' the 'good' bacteria for space in our guts. Subsequently, the LPS of these undesirable bacterial interlopers cause inflammation inside us, leading directly to obesity. [11]

Inflammation – a key cause of obesity

We know that when we injure ourselves, the area around the wound becomes red and inflamed. This is just our natural defence system doing its job in fighting off infection. However, this sort of inflammation happens inside our body as well, especially if we eat a high-sugar diet. Too much sugar feeds the bad bacteria and so upsets the balance of the bugs in our guts, particularly in the small intestine. This means we end up with increased numbers of 'bad' LPS circulating around our bodies, which in turn sets up an inflammatory response that leads directly to a number of health problems, such as increased risk of heart disease or cancer. Unfortunately, this sort of internal inflammation also leads directly to us becoming insensitive (or unresponsive) to both *insulin* and leptin. And, as we know, this sort of hormonal resistance lies at the heart of the obesity issue.

Good Calories, Bad Calories

When I started on my journey to find the answer to my ballooning weight, I soon became aware of the theory that obesity might be caused by excess carbohydrate consumption, leading to elevated insulin levels, leading in turn to *hyperinsulinaemia*, then *insulin resistance* and the subsequent storage of fat. This is discussed in the book *Good Calories, Bad Calories* by Gary Taubes. Not everyone agrees with this premise, but it goes like this:

"Carbs → excess insulin → hyperinsulinaemia → *insulin resistance* → obesity"

There are always two sides to a coin, of course, and other diet researchers have been quick to pour scorn on this slightly left-field theory. If I can be allowed to distill vast amounts of data and paperwork to one brief sentence, the other argument goes like this:

"Too many calories → obesity → *insulin resistance* →
hyperinsulinaemia"

Can you see the common denominator here? It doesn't matter how we spin it, insulin resistance is key to the current obesity epidemic. Regardless of whether or not Mr. Taubes is correct (I think he is), it is insulin resistance (and leptin resistance to a certain extent) that we need to address in order to rid ourselves of our obesity. Apart from the calories, something in our modern diet is causing us to be insulin and leptin resistant, which ultimately makes us fat.

Insulin resistance

Insulin and glucagon, the blood sugar hormones, are designed by evolution to fine-tune our blood sugar levels by giving them a mild tweak now and then after infrequent meals of real food – blood sugar levels are supposed to be fairly stable. However, with our modern, high-sugar diet, this fine-tuning goes out of the window.

Instead, we hammer our blood sugar levels all day long by constantly grazing on processed carbs (e.g. burger buns, breads, cakes, soft drinks, pies, pastries, chocolate bars, sweets and crisps). All our poor pancreas can do in response is unleash a tsunami of insulin in an attempt to stave off imminent hyperglycaemia. However, this unnaturally high level of insulin not only keeps us permanently in the 'fed' state, so we are constantly trying to store our food energy rather than use it, it also affects our ability to sense insulin in the first place.

And it's all to do with our genes. Our genes control everything and tell our bodies when to 'make something'. This includes making insulin receptors – those clever cellular structures that recognise insulin and allow the insulin molecule to 'dock' to the cell surface. However, if we bombard these receptors all day long with too much insulin, the genes that control their production get turned off, simply because our genes are trying to protect the cells from this unnaturally high level of insulin. We can soak up quite a lot of this excess insulin by exercising, probably because exercise uses glycogen that can be 'topped up' via the action of insulin without problem. However, if we are sedentary, the insulin in our bloodstream eventually causes our insulin receptor genes to shut down, leading directly to insulin resistance.[14]

Now we have a problem. At this point, more and more insulin has to be produced to achieve the same reduction in blood sugar concentration that used to be achieved by a much lower concentration of insulin, when we were insulin-sensitive. This overload of insulin eventually leads to *hyperinsulinaemia*[15, 16], a thoroughly undesirable condition with numerous consequences:

- High blood pressure (*hypertension*).
- Obesity.
- Inhibition of lipolysis ('fat burning').
- Inflammation (leading to higher risk of cardiovascular disease, strokes, cancers etc).
- Impaired glucose tolerance (this makes sense – too much glucose in the blood).
- Ageing?
- Worn-out pancreatic beta cells.
- Increased hunger, so we eat too much (via *hypoglycaemia*).
- Pre-disposition to type 2 diabetes.

How does insulin resistance relate to obesity? Well, this is a bit of a 'hot chestnut' because most scientists can't agree. Let's sum up it up as follows:

- Chronic (long-term) high levels of insulin in the blood will almost certainly lead to insulin resistance, which may lead to metabolic syndrome and, ultimately, type 2 diabetes. There is a connection between obesity and insulin resistance; however, this is a bit of a 'chicken and egg' scenario as it is not entirely clear whether obesity causes insulin resistance or whether insulin resistance leads to obesity.

I suspect there is probably a combination of the two in a sort of 'vicious circle'. Either way, this is yet another reason why we need to control our insulin levels as much as possible.

Type 2 diabetes – the ultimate 'disease of civilisation'?

If we keep eating the way we have been, we may well end up being unable to produce enough insulin to keep control of our blood sugar. In other words, we start to become *hyperglycaemic* and can no longer control that situation ourselves. Our pancreas also gets worn out by having to make excess insulin. At this point, a doctor will tell you that you have type 2 diabetes[17]. Your poor old insulin system has done its best, but our modern diet has defeated this remarkable control system. It's a bit like winning the Lottery, going out and buying a Ferrari and then leaving it in the garage with the engine running flat-out all day long, day after day. Eventually, something has to give.

Insulin is supposed to be produced in very small quantities after infrequent meals of natural, unprocessed foods, which allows our liver and muscle cells to remain acutely sensitive to the presence of insulin and respond accordingly. By contrast, our modern diet risks insulin resistance, with fairly disastrous consequences for our health.

Type 2 diabetes is a serious disease (with multi-factorial causes), requiring medical treatment from your doctor. I am not a medical doctor, nor a health professional, so if you have type 2 diabetes (or think you might have), please go and see your doctor in the first instance. He or she will look after you and monitor both your weight and your blood as you begin your diet. As a diabetic, you must speak to your doctor before embarking on this or any other diet. Diabetics take specific medication to control their blood sugar artificially, so there is a real danger of *hypoglycaemia* if sugar is suddenly stripped out of the diet while the drugs continue to be taken.

Nevertheless, I'm sure your doctor would be delighted if you were to lose weight, on this programme or any other. However, by following the Back to Basics diet in part two, I hope that those of you who might otherwise be on the 'conveyor belt' towards developing type 2 diabetes in the future will avoid doing so by regaining control of your waistline and your general health at the same time.

We don't need to eat all the time

Insulin and glucagon are supposed to 'tick away' in the background, ready to smooth out and stabilise blood sugar concentrations around infrequent meals of (very) low GI foods. However, our modern diet asks insulin to function much like the inexperienced captain of an extremely large boat. The captain turns the boat to starboard, but realises he has overdone it because the boat turns far more that he wanted. He spins the wheel the other way, only to find he has overcorrected again, leading to the ship swinging wildly to and fro either side of the intended course.

This is what happens to our insulin system when we eat frequent, high-sugar meals; unfortunately the rush of insulin can often remove too much glucose, resulting in a rather dramatic swing in blood sugar towards *hypoglycaemia*. We recognise the symptoms and, suddenly feeling woozy and unwell, we rush off for another high-sugar snack a few hours later. Insulin levels shoot back up, excess glucose is again swept out of the bloodstream and we are once more pushed towards *hypoglycaemia*. Eating high–sugar meals will inevitably lead to a wild swing in blood glucose levels (Fig 10).

The Back to Basics diet will help you calm all this down and allow the insulin/glucagon system to work correctly. By changing what we eat, together with making subtle changes to when we eat, we can regain control of our blood sugar levels and avoid the wild swings in blood sugar concentration that are so characteristic of our modern, high-sugar diet.

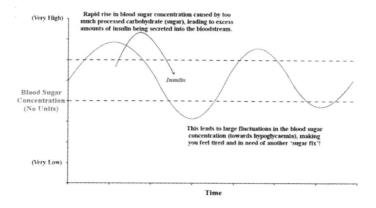

Fig 10. Fluctuations in blood sugar concentration caused by excess processed carbohydrate (and other rich foods).

Leptin, sensed in the hypothalamus of the brain, is our natural calorie counter. Leptin is supposed to curb our appetite by telling us when we are full and have eaten enough. However, much like insulin resistance, it seems that our modern diet makes us resistant to leptin[18], such that the hypothalamus does not recognise (or does not react to) the ever-increasing levels of leptin circulating in our ever-increasingly fat bodies.

I'm sure, like me, you know someone who seems able to eat what they want without putting on weight? To be fair, there will be a genetic component to their irritating slimness, but they will almost certainly be leptin-sensitive and we need to join them. So, by returning to a diet of real, natural foods and expunging sugar from our lives, we can begin to return our leptin system to normal levels of sensitivity. Then, much like our infuriatingly slim friends, we will sense when we are full and put down our knife and fork before we have eaten too many calories.

Regaining hormonal sensitivity on the Back to Basics programme

The Back to Basics programme is designed to achieve two key changes in your life. Firstly, by re-establishing a healthy relationship with food, you will be able to naturally reduce your calorie intake and so get your energy intake in balance once more. Secondly, the choice of foods, meal plans and particularly the timing of your meals is all about regaining sensitivity to insulin and leptin. As your hormonal sensitivity improves, you will instinctively eat fewer calories (thanks to leptin) and will be able to keep your insulin levels low as well. Not only will your calorie intake be under control, but you will also make much better use of your stored fat (via low insulin levels) and so will lose excess body fat rather than adding to it all of the time.

Chapter 6 summary:

- Many of us are intolerant to the processed carbohydrates in our modern diet – they are hard to digest, contain too many calories and make us fat.

- Real plant foods are actually low-carb due to the concept of carbohydrate density.

- Our modern, high-sugar diet favours the 'bad' bacteria in our guts that cause inflammation, leading to insulin and leptin resistance and obesity.

- Insulin resistance is at the heart of the obesity epidemic. To lose weight effectively, we simply must eat in a way that returns us to insulin sensitivity.

- Too much insulin in the bloodstream can lead to type 2 diabetes.

- Resistance to leptin means we lose control of our appetite and eat too much.

- We don't need to eat all of the time – our hormones are perfectly capable of managing our blood sugar levels on a real food diet.

- The Back to Basics diet will reduce your calorie consumption and return you to hormonal sensitivity.

7

Changing when we eat –
the final piece in the weight loss jigsaw

In this chapter, you will see why:

- Eating all of the time makes it impossible for us to lose weight.

- Our body chemistry can look after our blood sugar levels on its own, without us having to eat all the time.

- Changing when we eat will really help us to lose weight easily.

- Eating less often, in combination with plentiful activity, is the key to lifelong, effective weight loss.

I want to suggest a radically different approach to meal times. I know this may be controversial but changing *when* we eat, in combination with changing what we eat, is vital to permanent weight loss. If we alter the number, content and timing of our meals, we can use our body chemistry to best advantage, thus ensuring effective, permanent weight loss. This is a world away from the 'over-caloried' and 'insulinated' state we get ourselves into by eating all of the time.

Eat six meals a day? Not if you want to lose weight!

Why are you and I overweight? We are overweight because our modern diet contains too many calories and increases our insulin levels too much, too often. Excess calories obviously cause us problems, but too much insulin in the bloodstream also leads to obesity and insulin resistance – the start of the slippery slope towards lots of medical conditions as we have already seen.

Nevertheless, one of the most depressing pieces of dietary advice I have seen in the popular press and on the websites of certain so-called 'diet gurus' is the recommendation to eat five or six small meals every couple of hours throughout the day.[1] This, we are told, is necessary to keep our metabolism up so we can stabilise our blood sugar levels. I appreciate the sentiment but unfortunately, this advice is fundamentally wrong. If I haven't managed it so far, I hope I can convince you now that eating every couple of hours is certainly not how you or I are designed to eat[2].

Keeping our metabolism up?

What exactly is metabolism? It's a complicated subject but if you dig deep enough, you will find that metabolism is generally divided into two main categories: *catabolism* and *anabolism*[3].

We know these terms now, don't we? If you remember, *catabolism* is the breakdown and digestion of food to constituent parts (e.g. carbohydrate to glucose, fats to free fatty acids and glycerol and proteins to amino acids). In turn, *anabolism* is the process whereby these constituent parts are used to build up new cellular components, using the energy released during catabolism.

So, which metabolism will be used if we eat every couple of hours? The answer is catabolism, followed by anabolism. Uh oh, alarm bells! What is the main food hormone involved in anabolism? *Insulin.* So, by eating all of the time (six meals a day is definitely 'eating all of the time'), all we do is risk overeating calories and making ourselves permanently insulinated – both of which do tremendous damage to our waistlines and our health.

What about stabilising our blood sugar levels?

We know that our brain insists on a specific blood sugar (glucose) concentration, which roughly equates to one teaspoon of sugar in our total blood volume – which is not a lot of sugar. We are more than capable of keeping that level of blood sugar constant through our biochemistry and without the dubious benefit of constant eating, just as evolution worked out long ago. Although diabetics may have need for more frequent meals, it is a myth that the rest of us have to eat all the time to somehow manage our blood sugar levels – we are designed, by evolution, to function at our best on a lifestyle of daily activity and infrequent meals.[4] It will help us to lose weight if these infrequent meals are eaten at the same time each day, but eating all of the time is simply not necessary to control our blood sugar levels. In case you still don't believe me, let's take a closer look at how we can manage our blood sugar levels without stuffing our faces all of the time.

Our liver holds the key.

Imagine you have just woken up and got out of bed, ready for the new day. You haven't eaten for a while, so overnight your insulin levels have decreased. By definition therefore, your glucagon levels must be elevated. What does glucagon do? Well, amongst other things, glucagon encourages two complementary processes in the liver, both of which produce glucose to 'top up' your blood sugar to the correct level.[5] One process involves the breakdown of glycogen to glucose, known as *glycogenolysis*. The other process involves the production of new glucose from other non-carbohydrate 'bits' (such as amino acids, glycerol, lactate etc). This is known as *gluconeogenesis* – please don't worry about these science words!

So, when our blood sugar starts to drop during the night, the liver balances the breakdown of glycogen with the production of new glucose (if required), to keep our blood sugar level at the right concentration. It is a bit like the central heating thermostat in your house – you set a temperature you wish to be maintained (i.e. your blood sugar level) and the system turns the heating on and off as required to maintain that temperature. In our case, this control of our blood sugar is managed in the liver, mediated by insulin and glucagon. So, not only does a low insulin/high glucagon ratio enable us to burn away the fat from around our bodies so we lose weight, it keeps our blood sugar levels stable all of the time.

Do we really need to eat six meals a day?

So, how do six small meals a day 'smooth out' our blood sugar? It doesn't do anything of the sort, of course – it just forces us to burn glucose all the time, rather than the fat from the 'warehouse' around our bodies. And, unless we are very careful, we will eat too many calories and spend the whole day permanently insulinated as well. This is not the way to go about losing weight and regaining our health, I can assure you. So, please believe me when I say that we do *not* need to eat all of the time.

Changing *when* we eat to maximise low insulin levels

What's so wrong about having too much insulin in our bloodstream all day long? Well, if high levels of insulin block access to the tens of thousands of calories we have locked away in our fat (by inhibiting lipolysis); if it makes us add to our already bulging fat reserves all the time; if it makes us ill through inflammation, insulin resistance, type 2 diabetes and quite possibly shortens our lives by switching on the 'Grim Reaper' gene, surely it is common sense to minimise the time we spend insulinated as much as possible? Of course, if we have permanently raised insulin levels, it is very hard to lose weight as well – even with largely futile attempts at calorie counting or the occasional visit to the gym. [6]

However, a low level of insulin (or, if you like, a correspondingly high level of glucagon) allows us to manage our blood sugar levels quite happily and encourages lipolysis as well[7, 8]. We need to eat in such a way that we minimise our insulin response as much as possible – one way we can do this is by moving away from processed foods and returning to a predominantly vegetarian diet. Nevertheless, to get our insulin levels really under control, we are going to go further and change when we eat as well. This way, we can spend far more hours in the day in low insulin (when fat burning is optimised), rather than in a state of high insulin when our ability to lose weight is severely impaired. In so doing, we fit the final piece into the weight loss jigsaw and markedly improve our chances of lifelong, permanent weight loss. By tipping the odds in our favour this way, we will finally stop swimming against the tide of our own body chemistry.

The Back to Basics programme
will help you change when you eat

The Back to Basics programme will help you change when you eat so that you can keep your insulin levels at a low, background level for most of the day. This will help you regain insulin sensitivity; however, this doesn't mean we have to return to the Stone Age in order to eat correctly or return to a healthy weight. Simply by learning from these original human diets, we can make changes to *our* diet and lifestyle, including changing when we eat, to help us lose weight and improve our health as we return to a way of eating in accordance with our evolutionary design.

So, how exactly can we change when we eat in order to help us lose weight? Well, to get the ball rolling, imagine for a moment that we are looking at the clock face of a 24-hour clock (Fig 11).

Let's imagine you have just woken up at 7.00am after a good night's sleep. When did you last eat? That will have been when you had dinner at 7.00pm last night. So, what is going on with your insulin levels right now? Because you have been 'starving' through the night, your blood insulin levels are now low. Correspondingly, your blood glucagon levels are high and your liver will have kept your blood sugar levels 'topped up' through the night. However, what happens if our first act after getting up is to consume a high-carbohydrate, high-sugar breakfast (e.g. a bowl of cornflakes,

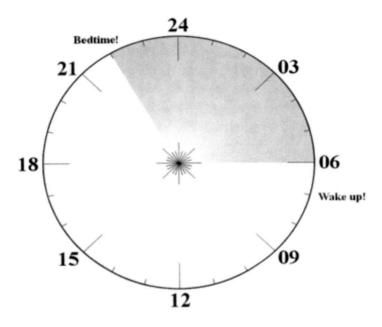

Fig 11. A 24-hour clock face.

some white bread toast with butter and marmalade)?

Well, everything changes! First of all, we unleash a tsunami of insulin from the pancreas in an attempt to remove all the excess sugar we have just dumped into our bloodstream from our sugary breakfast. Secondly, we risk sending our blood sugar levels yo-yoing up and down because such large amounts of insulin can sweep out too much glucose in one go, dropping us temporarily into hypoglycaemia. This drives us to consume sugary food again in order to balance our blood sugar – and off we go again! And it is very, very hard to lose weight when we are insulinated, as we now know.

Using daily activity to our best advantage

So, let's do something different. What do you think would happen if you gave breakfast a miss for a couple of hours and instead went out for a jog? Or cycled to work? Or walked the kids to school?

We know that when we wake up in the morning, insulin levels are low and glucagon levels are high. Remember the seesaw:

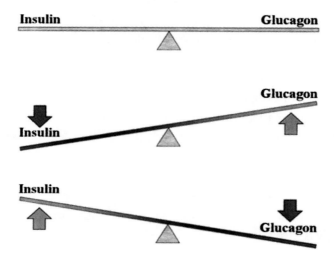

In our case, we have got out of bed and resisted the urge to eat something straightaway. Instead, we have pulled on our trainers and gone out of the front door. Once underway, we start to enjoy the outdoors, the fresh air and the wonderful sense of well-being that we get from taking activity. Before we realise it, we have walked, cycled or jogged for about forty-five minutes. This isn't a problem because today we got out of bed an hour earlier than usual, so we could get our morning fix of activity. Our heart rate monitor tells us that we have already used up 650 calories too, which means we are starting to improve our lives and lose weight as well. Happy days!

Where, though, is the energy coming from for this early morning activity? We haven't eaten breakfast yet, so we need to dip into our fuel reserves instead (i.e. glycogen and fat). This is all accessed quite naturally through our low insulin/high glucagon state, exactly how evolution has designed our bodies to work. By allowing our insulin levels to remain low at the beginning of the day, we are able to use our fuel reserves of fat and glycogen to provide loads of energy for even extended periods of activity.

Meanwhile, our blood sugar levels are taken care of by the breakdown of glycogen and, if necessary, a smidgen of gluconeogenesis – all controlled by the interplay of insulin and glucagon. Having returned from our morning excursion, we shower, get on our bike and cycle gently to work, burning a few more calories in the process. We are now free to enjoy a healthy breakfast or, better still, a brunch at some point later in the morning.

Living life in low insulin

Let's look at what have we achieved so far: we have taken most of our daily activity already and by not eating beforehand, we have worked *with* our body chemistry to access the stored energy from around our body – just as Nature intended. This early morning period, which I like to think of as the main 'low insulin' part of the day, is the ideal time to get active. This is also the time when we should not be eating. It is the time of day when we have naturally low insulin/high glucagon levels and so are primed to burn fat (i.e. lose weight), not store fat.

And now let's look at what happens when we eventually have something to eat: we now switch over to the 'fed' state and insulin once again regains the upper hand for a while. This is quite normal[9]. However, providing we only eat real food with a low GI (e.g. vegetables, berry fruits, lean meat/poultry, fish, eggs and healthy, natural fats in small quantities), we will not generate an excessive insulin response.

Instead, we will only require a small amount of insulin to smooth out our blood sugar levels – a few hours later, insulin will again take a back seat and glucagon levels will start to rise once more. This is what happened every day for millions of years whenever our *Paleo* ancestors ate something, before we messed it all up by over-processing food and discovering sugar.

Do you *really* want to get rid of that flab?

The more activity we take each day, the easier it will be for us to get our calorie intake in balance without having to eat small portions of food.[10] In other words, the more activity we do, the more calories we burn, so our normal portions of real food will contain (slightly) fewer calories than we expend. If we can manage our insulin levels as well, we are doing exactly what needs to be done to ensure we lose weight effectively. Having eaten a late(ish) breakfast or an early lunch (one or the other please – not both), our insulin levels should have returned to a background, low level by the afternoon – so can we now fit in some more activity?

Yes, because it is now time for our cycle ride home from work, our walk to collect the kids from school or our afternoon session at the gym. Once again, we are using our body chemistry to our advantage and are no longer swimming against the tide of insulin. By using our 'low insulin' phases of the day in this way, we are working with our body chemistry to access our stored energy (fat), rather than eating all the time and hence trying to lose weight in a permanent state of hyperinsulinaemia.

How many meals *should* we eat?

We are so accustomed to regarding three meals a day plus snacks as normal that any suggestion to eat less often is usually met with derision. However, we have already established that eating all of the time is unnecessary and potentially damaging to both our health and our waistlines, so how often should we eat? Well, as always in matters of human nutrition, there is no absolute answer. Nevertheless, to start with, I want you to try and give breakfast a miss. I appreciate this is controversial and I assure you I am not anti-breakfast as such; I just want you to break the habit of getting out of bed and immediately reaching for sugar in the form of breakfast cereal, white bread, pastries (croissants!), sugary tea and marmalade. Once you have done some activity in the morning, you can enjoy a late breakfast (or better still a brunch, which replaces both breakfast and lunch) of healthy, real foods, safe in the knowledge that you have taken a huge step towards a much healthier, slimmer way of life. Later, you can have a healthy snack of perhaps fruit or raw vegetables (about mid-afternoon), before looking forward to a delicious supper of healthy, tasty real foods.

We'll cover this in more detail in part two, but from now on, I would like you to think about just eating two meals a day (plus one mid-afternoon snack). Ideally, the first meal should be taken late in the morning or at lunchtime, after you have done some sort of morning activity – walking is fine. Your second meal should be taken in the early evening, again after some activity. You can have a snack of fruit or vegetables at some point in the afternoon. This may sound restrictive, but there is an enormous range of meals you can create around this template – and remember, I am not asking you to eat small portions. All we are trying to do is maximise the time we are best able to burn up our own fat as fuel (via low-insulin), while making sure that when we do eat, we eat plenty of highly nutritious, naturally low-calorie foods. This way, we will give ourselves the best possible chance of losing weight and keeping that weight off, long-term. Here is a suggested timetable for a typical day on the Back to Basics diet:

Alarm goes off	Time to get up!
Early morning	**ACTIVITY** – Walk to work, cycle to work, walk the kids to school, walk around the park.
Late morning / lunchtime	**EAT** – Time for the first meal of the day (one meal of healthy, nutritious, predominantly vegetarian food). Take a packed brunch to work.
Mid-afternoon	**SNACK** – Fruit, vegetables, hummus?
Late afternoon	**ACTIVITY** – Walk home from work, cycle home from work, walk the kids back from school, walk around the park.
Early evening	**EAT – Time for dinner.** Eat at the table and enjoy a glass of wine.

Eat your meals to suit *your* lifestyle

Nothing is set in stone and you should use common sense in terms of your own meal times. Work your mealtimes around your particular lifestyle, as the time of day you eat is less important than the number and content of meals you eat in total – provided you eat at the same time each day. For instance, if you get up at dawn and then do two or three hours of hard labour (a farmer, for instance), you might eat your breakfast before 9.00am. On another day, you might have a lie–in, then get up and go for a walk or go to the gym or go for a bike ride and so not eat much before your normal lunchtime. In both cases, you are playing by the rules because activity comes before eating. This just keeps us in our overnight low insulin phase as long as possible before we 'break our fast'; in so doing, we give ourselves the best chance of burning fat before we start to consume calories once again.

Personally, I eat my first meal of the day at lunchtime, then have a mid-afternoon snack of fruit or crudities and an early supper, often one of my 'Wonder Salads' plus some healthy protein. This helps me control my eating and allows me to take my daily activity when I am naturally in a state of low insulin. I recommend you do the same but we'll cover this in more detail in part two.

Intermittent fasting –
Nature's natural weight control

What I am proposing here (changing when we eat to maximise weight loss) is my interpretation of something known in the trade as *intermittent fasting* (IF). Numerous diets employ 'IF' to some degree or another, but as always in the field of human nutrition, there are as many people opposed to fasting as there are supporters of it. All I ask is that you give my version of 'IF' a go, as it is based on sound biochemical principles and will really help you in your quest to lose weight. [11, 12, 13]

The Back to Basics diet will help you change the way you eat to make best use of low blood insulin levels. This just means you have to plan your meals (a bit), so that you maximise your body's ability to burn fat, which is, after all, what we are trying to do. From now on, just try and squeeze your eating into a smaller period of the day, rather than switching your insulin system on first thing in the morning with a sugary breakfast and then keeping it high all day long by grazing on processed food and junk food. With a bit of practice, you will soon be able to forego your sugary breakfast immediately on rising and replace it with some morning activity. After that, you will be free to have a healthy, nutritious, low-calorie breakfast a bit later.

With a bit more practice, you can delay this late breakfast by an hour or two and turn it into a brunch instead. This way, you can really start to maximise your ability to lose weight. By squeezing all of your eating into a six or seven-hour period of the day, you only spend a few hours each day gently insulinated and then spend far more hours in a state of low insulin, burning fat. In so doing, you will return to a way of life that evolution has designed us to follow. So, just like our *Paleo* ancestors, you will become slim, fit and a lot happier, too. Sounds like a plan to me.

Chapter 7 summary:

- Eating all of the time is not the way to lose weight.

- Our body chemistry can easily manage our blood sugar levels without us having to eat all of the time.

- Changing when we eat puts the final piece into the weight-loss jigsaw.

- Eating less often, plus getting active twice a day, is the key to lifelong, effective weight loss.

8

Summing it all up

Where has it all gone wrong?

Ever since the Industrial Revolution, we in the West have migrated from the farmlands to towns and cities in search of a better life and the higher wages associated with an industrial society. Unfortunately, this has led to a complete change in the way we all eat. Having left the world of subsistence agriculture behind, food now had to be produced on a massive scale, requiring a level of food processing never before seen in human history. On top of all this, we have been told for decades to eat a low-fat, high-carbohydrate diet, leading to a huge increase in the consumption of processed carbohydrate. Since the 1960s or thereabouts, we have also had the 'double whammy' of sugar (e.g. HFCS) being added to myriad processed foods and a simultaneous explosion in the fast food culture, which is now so popular around the globe.

Add all this together and what have we got? A society that perceives normal eating as the constant grazing of calorie-rich, but nutritionally poor, processed carbohydrate foods coupled to reduced levels of activity. Result? Inflammation, insulin resistance, leptin resistance, the massive overeat of calories and a worldwide epidemic of obesity.

Our modern Western diet – the 'conveyor belt' to obesity

We know that our obesity is not our fault, so why do we really get fat? Is it just down to the calories in our food? Is it all about inflammation, insulin resistance and leptin resistance? Or is it simply about the types of food in our diet today? I'm sure the reason we get fat is down to some dastardly combination of all of the above. But do you know what? It just doesn't matter.

Let the doctors and scientists argue over the technical pathways that link our modern diet to obesity – all we need to understand is that our old diet of processed carbs, too much fat and sugar (Fig 12) not only gave us too many calories for little benefit, but also upset our body chemistry such that it was almost impossible to resist putting on weight. Surely, that is enough to make us dump our modern diet and return to eating the way we are designed to eat?

Our weight is ultimately controlled by the balance of the calories we eat, compared to the calories we use up each day of our lives. Nevertheless, by simply saying, "eat less and move more", the dietary establishment has attempted to cure the worldwide obesity epidemic in a completely ineffective manner. By contrast, we have gone to great lengths to work out *why* we eat too many calories and why the highly

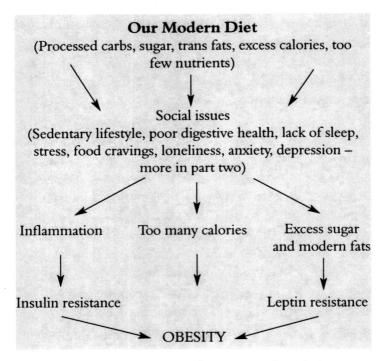

Fig. 12 Our modern diet – the root cause of our obesity.

calorific foods we eat today cause us to switch over to storing fat all the time and make it hard for us not to overeat or otherwise make ourselves ill. Simply eating less modern food will never work. We now know that the secret to healthy, lifelong weight loss involves eating fewer calories through a return to a natural, predominantly vegetarian diet, which supplies us with lots of wonderful nutrients for relatively few calories and gives our hormones a rest.

Over to you

Here, then, at the end of part one, I want to invite you to change your life. In a moment, you will discover all the wonderful, real foods that are going to make up your new, healthy diet. There is no place here for processed food, junk food or any man-made rubbish that makes us both ill and fat. Instead, we will rediscover the wonderful world of real food – what it consists of, how we should source it, how we should prepare it and how we can enjoy it for the rest of our lives, while becoming healthy, happy and slim along the way.

Seems like a pretty good reason to read part two to me!

Summary of the Back to Basics Diet so far:

- Being overweight or obese is not your fault.

- Our modern diet contains too many calories for little nutritional benefit. It also disturbs certain hormones (insulin and leptin) in such a way that we find it very hard not to overeat and spend far too much time trying to store fat, rather than using our body fat to power our lives.

- Yes, we have to eat fewer calories than we burn in order to lose weight. However, if we change the type of foods we eat, in conjunction with controlling when we eat (all in part two), the calories will look after themselves.

- Our evolutionary history has designed us to eat a predominantly vegetarian diet, together with natural (organic) meat, fish and fat.

- Our modern, high-sugar diet not only contains unnecessary calories, but also leads directly to insulin and leptin resistance. This is the underlying cause of much of the obesity epidemic and the basis of the various 'diseases of civilisation' we see all around us today.

- Our modern, high-sugar diet leads to inflammation inside our bodies (quite probably via our 'bad' gut bacteria), which not only increases our risk of developing many nasty diseases, but also leads, again, to insulin and leptin resistance.

PART TWO

Getting to grips with the Back to Basics Diet

9

It's time to put you first for a change!

*Our greatest glory is not in never falling,
but in getting up every time we do.*
Confucius

Welcome to part two of the Back to Basics diet programme. Everything you need to complete your journey to a new, healthier, happier, slimmer version of you is here, including diet plans, tips and recipes. However, before we launch into the plan itself, I just want to talk for a moment about you – the most important part of this whole story.

It's time to look after Number One!

I know from bitter experience how easy it is to lose control of our relationship with food. As that relationship starts to fall apart, our self-confidence and self-esteem hit rock bottom and we get ever more demoralised and depressed. We find every excuse in the book to avoid changing our diet and lifestyle and often become morose and irritated with those around us who are trying to help, even though they invariably have our best interests at heart. Does this ring a bell? Well, that's all in the past. From now on, I want you to completely rethink your attitude to food and exercise, so that before doing anything else on each day of your life, you consider *your* needs first.

I also reckon it's a pretty safe bet to say that for far too long, you have run yourself into the ground and have ignored your own health and happiness? So, from now on, I want you to think about your meals and your daily routine first, before anything else, each and every day. It's time to put your health and happiness first for a change. I know this goes against every fibre of your being, but if you want to lose weight (I mean *really* lose weight) you need to look after Number One.

Are you too busy to bother about food?

I can hear you now: "What about the kids? I have to get the children to school! What about my family's meals? I have a full-time job! How on earth am I supposed to find the time to go food shopping or cook proper meals?"

We all have responsibilities in life, but stop and think for a moment about why you have put on weight. You have probably gained weight through eating too many calories, coupled to sending your food hormones haywire from a lifetime of eating too much processed food and sugar. But more importantly, you have gained weight because you have failed to put yourself first in life. You have stopped thinking about *your* food and *your* health on a daily basis, and so have lost control of sensible eating habits. Unfortunately, this all ends up as the slippery slope to obesity and ill health. It is precisely because we are 'too busy to bother' that we grab something on the go, or pick up a takeaway on the way home from work. Yes, we are all busy. Yes, to eat healthily takes a bit of planning and organisation. But think of the alternative? I know you want to change your life because you have made the effort to get hold of this book. Good for you, you are halfway there.

However, to really make that transition to a new, healthy you, you are going to have to go further. Just for a few weeks or at least until it becomes second nature, I want you to be selfish. I want you to think about *your* daily routine, *your* food and *your* meals before everything else. Even before family, career, friends, you need to realise that 'what am I going to have for lunch and dinner' is the most important decision of each and every day. Only by putting yourself first in this way can you learn to regain control of your eating and exercise habits. Once you are off and running, by all means include your family and friends in your new healthy lifestyle. However, for now, it is all about you.

It is time to change your life for the better

For this to work, you are going to have to accept that in some ways, your life is about to change. Changing something at our stage in life is hard, but that doesn't mean it is not worth attempting or impossible to do. What matters is that we do something *now* about our weight, before it is too late. My father used to joke about a pub he frequented in London in the 1950s, which had a permanent sign on the bar saying 'Free Beer Tomorrow!' As we know, tomorrow never comes. So, we need to act now, today, by changing to a whole new, healthy way of life. This is what the Back to Basics diet programme is all about – helping *you* to change to a new, slim, healthy version of you.

All I ask is a commitment to change – to change your mindset and to change your way of living, shopping, cooking and taking activity. Yes, you probably will have to make some changes to your lifestyle, but as in most things in life, something that is worth the reward will invariably require some effort and sacrifice along the way. I just want you to accept that you have to be selfish for a little while, for your own sake.

The Back to Basics Diet will help you take care of yourself

Although changing the way you eat might feel awkward and unnatural at first, losing weight on this programme does not depend on you eating tiny portions of food or otherwise using willpower to resist your natural hunger pangs. Most diets fail because the dieter eventually gets so hungry, he or she can no longer ignore the natural human instinct to eat. However, that won't happen here because I am only asking you to change *what* you eat and *when* you eat, rather than restricting food quantity, so you will never feel deprived or hungry. Within reason, you can eat as much food as you like – provided you stick to the rules.

Nothing is more important than your health and happiness. Remember, you owe it to yourself, your family and loved ones to finally accept that *you* are the most important part of this story. It is *your* health that has to come first.

Happy? Good, let's move on.

10

Breaking old habits

You may have heard the expression, 'it only takes twenty-one days to change a habit'? Well, that's fine, but I think we should all be prepared to invest a bit more time and effort in adjusting to a new, healthier diet and lifestyle. You are going to have to make some significant changes to your diet and lifestyle on the Back to Basics programme, but I will help you with that – don't worry! Nevertheless, this is a million miles away from the much-discredited idea of going on a diet. Instead, I want you to use my programme as a template for life, a system to be used in the short term for weight loss and then as a lifelong framework for rebuilding a much healthier version of you in the years ahead.

Willpower? Not needed here!

You don't need me to tell you how hard it is to stick to a traditional diet. We begin full of good intentions, only to find after a couple of weeks that the wheels fall off and we return to the comfort of our old ways. You and I are not alone – millions of well-intentioned people fall off the wagon like this every year, even though they are just as desperate to lose weight as we are. The main problem on most diets is that we are expected to eat very small portions of food; this means that we have to use huge amounts of willpower just to resist our desire to eat more food. Sure, we will lose weight in the short term, but because the meals are so small, we will soon get hungry and no amount of willpower will resist our urge to eat. If the diet also involves weird, expensive or obscure ingredients, it is highly unlikely that we will stick with it for any length of time either.

Unfortunately, diets just don't work

If we try to lose weight by eating tiny portions of food, we will just end up back at square one, I'm afraid. Despite the plethora of fad diets that exist today, any form of food restriction is doomed to failure because we can never resist our innate desire to eat. So, how is the Back to Basics diet different? We *are* going to change the way we eat so that we are once again in accord with our evolutionary design, but this does not mean we have to return to living in caves. Yes, we do need to reduce our calorie consumption, but we can achieve this quite easily through a diet of plentiful, delicious, fresh, healthy, real food.

By basing our meals around fairly large portions of vegetables, salads and fruit, we can fill ourselves up and get vastly more micronutrients (e.g. vitamins, minerals and phytonutrients) than we have had in a long time. We will no longer be crying out for nutrients all the time and will finally be in control of our appetites. In fact, much of what we call hunger is just sugar and micronutrient cravings, neither of which are ever truly satisfied with a high-calorie, low-nutrient modern diet.

We just need a little willpower to change

So, where does willpower fit into the Back to Basics programme? The only willpower I want you to call upon is in helping you to *change*; changing how you eat, changing from your old habits to embracing my plan, changing and organising your daily routine, changing your shopping habits and changing your whole life by committing – really committing – to following the plan. You will then be off and running; your cravings will ease and you will not require any particular willpower to stick to the programme for the rest of your life.

Getting active everyday

I bet you were hoping I would forget all about exercise, weren't you? Unfortunately, there is no getting away from it. As well as changing what and when we eat, if we want to lose weight and improve our health we are going to have to take some exercise as well. The good news is that from now on, I will use the much more friendly term 'activity'. Getting active everyday is central to the Back to Basics diet, so it is time to face those demons and accept that we need to break one of our most ingrained habits – the habit of being sedentary.

Have you tried to exercise in the past but lost heart because it made you feel uncomfortable or self-conscious and, anyway, it made no difference to your waistline? I sympathise; like you, I struggled to shift any weight by exercising until I worked out how to change my relationship with food as well. Although I am now quite active and love my skiing, hill walking and scuba diving, I didn't really begin to lose any weight until I changed my eating habits (as per this programme) in combination with taking up *daily* activity. Quite understandably, most of us today have lost sight of what constitutes normal levels of human activity (i.e. the level of exercise you and I are designed, by evolution, to take). This is certainly the case if we compare the amount of activity we take in our day-to-day lives, compared to how active our *Paleo* ancestors were, or how active any number of Aboriginal peoples around the World are today.

What is the best form of activity? It's called 'Life'!

As nutrition blogger Stephan Guyenet once said, " Our ancestors had a different word for exercise – Life!" This sums up our problem in a nutshell; our ancestors, the Kitavans, the peasants on the Island of Crete in the 1950s etc all had a lifestyle that involved almost *constant* activity, often involving hard physical effort and manual labour in just about every one of their waking hours. Not only did they burn oodles of calories, but they also developed wonderfully healthy, strong bodies, too.

So, where does our twice-weekly trip to the spinning class at the gym fit into this story? Well, it is certainly better than nothing! Nevertheless, if we then spend the rest of the week doing no exercise at all, we are not really making any difference to our long-term health. Instead, we need to take some tips from these happy, more traditional peoples and try to change our whole attitude to activity on a *daily* basis.

Learning to walk all over again

So, what is the best way to start getting active everyday? Well, there are a number of options, but first of all I want you to learn to walk all over again! Of course, we all know how to walk, don't we – we have been doing it since we were toddlers. Even so, how many of us actually walk any distance each day? We have become so programmed to using the car, catching the bus or getting on the train that very few of us walk any distance at all. So, what's the big deal about walking?

It seems that our earliest human ancestors did not suffer from obesity or many other modern diseases, such as cancer and heart disease. To be blunt, fat people would not have survived for very long in those days because they would have literally 'fallen by the wayside' and been left for dead. So, how did they stay slim? We know they ate a diet of real, unprocessed, predominantly vegetarian foods, supplemented by relatively infrequent meals of meat or fish, but they were also constantly active. Did our ancestors have annual gym membership? Did the Neanderthals invent Lycra®? Of course not! They stayed slim because they *walked*, a lot.

Walking is our natural daily activity

Back in *Paleo* times, every waking moment would have been taken up with a list of simple priorities – to find water, find food, find shelter, stay alive and reproduce. Life wasn't terribly complicated in those days. All of this involved a lot of walking (well, perhaps not reproduction!) because *every* calorie was precious. Daily life was measured in costs; costs in foraging for food, costs in time, costs in risking being eaten by a predator and costs in being attacked by another tribe. Do you think our ancestors would have spent all day running marathons? Most unlikely – why waste calories? Yes, they would have pursued game for extended periods, but they would have mostly walked and perhaps sprinted a few hundred yards for the kill.

Similarly, they would have walked until attacked by a predator, then sprinted to get away before dropping back to a walk once again. Calories had to be preserved. All this walking would have kept them very fit (and without the damage to joints and back that can occur from too much jogging) and would have kept obesity at bay, too. To our eyes, these people would have appeared very lean, but they would

still have had enough body fat to see them through periods
of famine.

We are designed to walk

One of the most important changes that happened in our
evolution from ape to Man was when we 'stood up' and
started to walk on our hind legs. We are *meant* to walk.
Walking requires no special equipment and can be easily
included into our daily life. So, from now on, get yourself
some trainers and just go out of your front door and walk.
How fast should you walk? I think the fitness professionals
suggest you keep to a pace that allows you to hold a
conversation. Swing your arms, get a bit of a glow on and
enjoy the fresh air. Keep safe (avoid busy main roads and
remote parks after dark) and just enjoy it. Walking is fun; if
you want to be sociable, get your friends and family to walk
along with you. We are talking about changing your lifestyle
for good, which means you need to be active *every* day.
Walking is by far and away the best and easiest way to start
getting active every single day.

As always, please go and see your GP before you start,
just to make sure all is well before you hit the streets.
Although I recommend you start getting active through
walking, if you would prefer to cycle then by all means get
on your bike instead. If you like swimming, go swimming
everyday. It's entirely up to you – just get active everyday.
Here are some suggestions for building activity into *your* day:

GETTING ACTIVE EVERYDAY

- Catch the bus to work? Walk instead.
- Pushed for time? Walk to the bus stop a mile down the road, not the one outside your front door.
- Walk the kids to school and back home again in the afternoon.
- Go for a walk around the park at lunchtime, rather than sitting idly in the staff canteen and stuffing your face with processed food.
- Take the kids for a walk around the park after school or get a dog and walk him twice a day, every day.
- Have to be in the office by 9.00am? Set your alarm an hour earlier and cycle to work, rather than using the car. Obviously, you have to cycle home at the end of the day, too.
- Join a walking/cycling club, go hiking in the hills at weekends, go for a walk before getting the kids ready for school, go out for a bike ride for pleasure etc.
- Find something that suits you – staying on the couch is not an option.

Get the idea? Each and every one of us has a different lifestyle and although we all go about our lives in a similar way, we all have different priorities and personal circumstances. We just need to look at our own daily routine to find ways to build activity into our new, healthy lifestyle

Are you still too busy?

"But I'm too busy, Dave", you cry. "I've got a business to run; it's a nightmare to get the kids ready for school; I have to go to work, do the shopping, cook dinner etc." OK, you are busy, but what did we say before about looking after Number One? Unless you put your own health and happiness first, nothing will change. You have to make some time for you from now on, which includes working out how you can make time for your chosen daily activity. All it takes is a bit of planning and reorganisation.

Once you have got the ball rolling, you can encourage your family and friends to join you in becoming active, too. When they see you losing weight, getting fitter and obviously becoming much happier in life, they will want to join you. Introduce them to this book (sorry, shameless commercial plug!) and get them to join you as you lose weight and develop your fitness. It is a win–win situation.

Taking things further

If you want to take things further, there is plenty of help out there in the form of websites, gyms and personal trainers. However, if you are currently sedentary (nobody is looking over your shoulder, so be honest with yourself) and haven't done any exercise for a long time, then you need to start off nice and slow (i.e. by learning to walk in the first instance). You will enjoy it once you get going and will have far more success in losing weight and keeping it off than if you steadfastly remain a couch potato. Just remember to check with your GP before you pull on that tracksuit.

If you want to do more, just remember that nobody is going to bully you into doing something that hurts or is generally unpleasant – least of all me. I want you to discover the joy of becoming active again for yourself, without fear of being laughed at or humiliated or otherwise made to suffer. I have been there and it is not a pleasant experience. So, when you are ready, by all means get yourself down to the local gym and link up with a personal trainer if you wish – many municipal gyms offer this service for free. Just remember we are talking about getting active everyday, so perhaps workouts are best left until later when you have got used to getting out and about in the fresh air, for a few weeks at least.

Nevertheless, if you want to take things beyond walking, that's great! Get a bicycle, take up a sport, learn a martial art, go swimming and play tennis – just be careful not to overdo it in the early weeks and months of your new regime. If you are very heavy or otherwise very new to any form of activity, I strongly suggest you stick to walking until you have lost some weight and have started to develop some basic fitness. After that, the world's your oyster! Please remember to check with your doctor before commencing your chosen form of activity – just be sensible.

Calories in – calories *out*

This leads me neatly onto a final discussion about the dreaded calorie. At the beginning of the book, I explained that to lose weight we needed to consume fewer calories than we burn up. The Back to Basics diet helps us with this because the foods you are going to eat are naturally low-calorie.

Nevertheless, it would make life much easier all round if we worked on the other side of the 'calories in – calories out' equation, too. Remember that our Basal Metabolic Rate (BMR) gives us the number of calories we need to stay alive under normal conditions (see Appendix 1 for BMR sum). If you follow the recommended eating plans in this programme, you will find it hard to eat much more than your BMR each day anyway. Obviously, if you are very large, you may have a larger BMR and you might need to eat a bit more along the way; nevertheless, any activity we can do above and beyond our BMR will tip the 'calories in – calories out' equation in our favour. So, if we burn up more calories than we eat, our body will have to find those extra calories from somewhere else. Any guesses where? From glycogen and our fat. And if we minimise the time we spend insulinated, we will make it *much* easier for our body to access this fat for fuel.

Use a heart rate monitor to see those calories disappear

Once you are in the habit of getting active everyday and are ready to take things further, I strongly suggest you save up and invest in a heart rate monitor. This is a simple and relatively cheap piece of sports equipment, popular with athletes and runners, which you can buy at most sports shops or online for approximately £30. You have to do a bit of setting up before you start (input your age, sex and weight) and after that, the 'brain' in the watch does the rest.

This clever gadget records your heart rate very accurately and as you start to huff and puff, the 'brain' calculates how many calories you are using, as well as keeping track of time and training zones for your heart rate. Remember that *any* activity will burn calories, so try this as a bit of a trick – put your heart rate monitor on in the morning and set off to work. It is very discreet under your clothes, so nobody will know! Try and walk to work or at least a part of the way there. Use the stairs, not the lift. Go for a walk at lunchtime. All the while, keep an eye on your monitor and see how many calories you have burned. You will very quickly adjust your daily activity to suit you, and as you see the calories getting burned each day, you will get more and more inspired to become ever more active. In this way, you will be well on your way to being as fit and as trim as you have been in years. Go for it!

11

*Learning to re-establish a
healthy relationship with food*

The Back to Basics programme is designed to achieve
effective weight loss over the long term through a sensible
diet of *real* food. So, before we launch into the
programme itself, perhaps we should take a few moments
to look at all the wonderful, tasty, nutritious and healthy
foods we are going to eat (and fall in love with) in our
new, healthy life. The Back to Basics diet will introduce
you to:

- A wonderful variety of real, natural foods that will help
  you lose weight and boost your health.

- The idea of eating fruit and vegetables *in season* – I want
  you to embrace real, natural foods in their normal
  growing cycle to maximise your health and minimise
  our impact on the planet.

- Some ideas about how to source real, natural proteins in
  your diet.

- Ways to eat oils and fats in sensible quantities on a perfectly healthy diet.

So, what *are* we going to eat?

I nearly called this chapter 'what we can't eat', but I thought that sounded far too depressing. So, in the spirit of our newfound enthusiasm for a healthy diet, I have decided to concentrate on all the wonderful foods we can eat in abundance instead. Let's now turn the spotlight on the enormous array of nutritious, tasty, natural foods that are going to form the basis of your Back to Basics diet. These foods are relatively cheap to buy and abundantly available and once you start to embrace these foods as part of your new life, you will soon find that they are a delight to eat and easy to make into a huge variety of delicious meals.

Stick to local, real foods

The Back to Basics diet does *not* require any obscure or weird ingredients – you know the ones, found growing on a rare tree in the Himalayas and picked at dawn by a virgin on a Tuesday when the moon is full. OK, I am being silly, but many fad diets do ask us to search out the most bizarre and obscure foods imaginable. These foods might well be available in a hippy commune in Southern California, but as sure as eggs are eggs, you and I are not going to find them in our local supermarket. This is yet another reason why many diets fail in the long term, so everything that follows here is about learning to seek out and choose the right foods from our usual local suppliers. Most of these foods have been staring us in the face for years, but we have just walked right past them on our way to the ready meals or the takeaway counter.

No specialist cooking skills required!

I am just a typical English bloke, but despite this, I am quite an enthusiastic cook. In fact, I suspect that many of my weight issues stemmed from me spending too much time in my own kitchen, where I enthusiastically embraced the 'quick slurp' school of male cookery. In the privacy of my own kitchen, it was all too easy to down a couple of glasses of wine and graze on numerous savoury snacks while tending to my gastronomic masterpiece. Consequently, I could easily reach my calorie allowance for the day before sitting down to eat my dinner. So, beware the nibbles and the bottle of wine in the fridge.

Nevertheless, you will not have to spend all day in the kitchen preparing complicated meals on the Back to Basics programme, unless you really want to. Later, I will introduce some simple meal ideas, made from real, tasty food, which you can prepare in double-quick time. This means you don't have to spend hours toiling away in the kitchen where temptation lies in wait. You won't need to enroll on a professional chef's course either, to enjoy eating this type of food. However, if you love cooking and feel that it would help you come to terms with your new diet by playing around with recipes and creating more elaborate meals, then please be my guest. Just remember to stick to the rules, as explained in the programme coming up.

The foods of the Back to Basics Diet

What follows now is a quick gallop through the types of food you are going to meet in the recommended diet plans coming up. I am assuming that you have read the preceding chapters of the book and so are reasonably happy with some of the main concepts we have covered so far (e.g. the need to eat a predominantly vegetarian diet, only eating real food, carbohydrate density, the dangers of processed foods and sugar etc). If any or all of these ideas are still unclear, then just flick back through the earlier chapters from time to time so you can refresh your memory. I have not included any recipes here, but you will find some suggestions for meal plans and recipes at the back of the book.

So, let's look at all of the wonderful foods that are going to form the basis of our diet from now on. I will look at each food category from a UK shopping and home cooking perspective, but the basic principles apply to all of us – regardless of where we live.

Good carbs – fruit and vegetables

Many of us have a dislike of vegetables, often going back to experiences in childhood. Nevertheless, if we want to lose weight effectively *and* become healthy, we have to face our demons and make eating some fruit and *lots* of vegetables the central part of each and every meal. There is no getting away from it, I'm afraid. We will look at fruit in a moment, so let's just think about vegetables for now.

We know that our evolutionary history has designed us to function at our best on a predominantly vegetarian diet, but what does this mean in reality? Should we just have an extra Brussels sprout at Christmas? Do we *have* to eat the token salad atop our takeaway burger and fries? Sorry, not even close.

I used this phrase earlier in the book: 'We are eating in a way that is completely out of kilter with our evolutionary design'. Well, the simplest way to redress our 'out of kilter' diet is to replace all of the processed carbohydrate with fruit and lots of salad and vegetables. Because of the idea of carbohydrate density, this type of real plant food is actually low-carb, and is naturally low in calories but very high in nutrients (i.e. quite unlike processed carbohydrate). By eating lots of real plant foods, we can reverse the damage of a lifetime, start to lose weight effortlessly and painlessly, and boost our health and happiness all in one fell swoop.

Why eat plants?

The evidence from some of the World's leading scientists is now pretty unequivocal; levels of fruit and vegetable consumption are intimately associated with rates of heart attacks, strokes and cancer (see bibliography for multiple references). In other words, the *more* fruit and vegetables you eat, the *less* chance you have statistically of developing any or all of these nasty conditions or diseases. We simply have to come to terms with the fact that long-term weight loss and overall health is fundamentally linked to the quantity of fruits and vegetables in our diet. It is as simple as that; fruits and vegetables truly *are* the panacea to our long-term health.

Such remarkable health benefits are mainly down to the number and variety of phytochemicals contained in plants. These wonderful, naturally occurring chemicals are contained in fruits, salad and vegetables in large amounts and in enormous variety. Scientists are only just beginning to identify the chemical structure of some of these substances and are light years away from ever identifying the whole range of beneficial chemicals found in plants.

Yet again, Nature has come up with the perfect solution to human health, if only we would take the time to see what is in front of our eyes. There are literally thousands of plants (and associated fruits) of all shapes, sizes and colours on this planet of ours, so it is high time we included just *some* of these 'wonder foods' in our diet.

Try to eat fresh food in season as much as you can

I appreciate that food is generally expensive nowadays, but fruit and vegetables need not cost the Earth. Ideally, we should grow our own – a polytunnel at home or a local allotment is *the* new status symbol in life. Failing that, try and buy fruits and vegetables locally and in season. That means that in the UK, we should not be eating strawberries at Christmas or Brussels sprouts in July.

In these enlightened times, there is no excuse for not supporting local growers and farmers and enjoying their wonderful, fresh, seasonal produce throughout the year. Not only is this healthier and cheaper for us, but it keeps our carbon footprint low and is good for the planet as well.

So, it is time to put aside our childish objections to healthy eating and look at fruits and vegetables in a completely different light. The Back to Basics diet will give you a detailed, structured eating plan to help you make the transition from the 'old you', who probably didn't eat many vegetables, to the fantastic, slim, healthy, happy 'new you', who eats lots of vegetables! By changing to a predominantly vegetarian diet, you will not only give yourself the best chance of successful long-term weight loss, but will also vastly improve your ability to preserve and enhance your health for the rest of your life. Replacing the processed carbohydrate and junk food with fresh fruits and vegetables is central to this programme, so by making this simple change to your diet, you will be able to lose weight *and* boost your health and sense of well-being to a whole new level.

Fruit

In his book *Fit for Life*, Sir Ranulph Fiennes states, "Fruit is truly the panacea to good health." He's right and fresh fruit will certainly form a very important part of our new, healthy diet in the future. However, certain fruits are very high in sugar (fructose, mostly), so we just need to be a little careful about how much fruit we eat in the early stages of our new, real food diet, particularly if we are diabetic or pre-diabetic –medical conditions that should be checked for you by your doctor. So, I recommend sticking to fruits that are not particularly sweet at first, such as the berries (e.g. raspberries, blueberries, strawberries, loganberries, blackberries, tayberries etc).

However, for most of us, the benefits of eating fruit massively outweigh the risk that a small amount of natural fructose might have on our health. Nevertheless, if you are diabetic, you might be best advised to avoid fruits altogether until your blood sugar levels are better controlled. As always, please ask your doctor for specific advice. For the rest of us, lots of fruit will do us the world of good.

OK, let's leave fruit and vegetables for now and look at the other foods we can eat on the Back to Basics diet.

Choosing protein on the Back to Basics Diet

It is time to give up all those man-made ready meals and takeaways that made us fat and unhealthy and switch to eating real, natural foods instead. This includes our proteins, such as meat and fish. You won't be eating a lot of these foods, as vegetables will make up about 80% of each meal, so you will be saving money on this programme as well. As a result, it is well worth seeking out good quality proteins; today, it is fairly easy to find healthy poultry and fish in the supermarket, local shops or online. To help you on your way, I have listed some recommended suppliers at the end of the book. From now on, try and eat these types of foods as your main source of protein (and other nutrients) on the Back to Basics diet:

- **Meat** – Try and source organic meat as much as possible and only eat meat in *limited* quantities (i.e. once or twice a week at most). As a happy by-product, eating meat infrequently saves a lot of money! Try organic beef, pork, lamb or better still, wild venison.

- **Poultry** – Find a good source of local, organic chicken etc. They need not be too expensive and can easily be made to feed a family for two, if not three, meals (more later).

- **Fish** – Finding high-quality, ethically-sourced fish can be a bit of a minefield, but the situation is definitely improving – at least in the UK. I recommend you eat lots of fish, because so long as we are careful in our choices, fish is a healthy and highly nutritious foodstuff and an excellent source of protein. Certain fish also provide high levels of very beneficial Omega 3 fatty acids.

- **Eggs** – A natural human food. Source high-quality, free-range organic eggs (or keep your own chickens?) and enjoy a few times each week.

- **Dairy** – We are only designed to consume *one* type of dairy product: our mother's milk. We are *not* designed to consume the milk of other mammals and, in particular, the milk from cows. I do use a little skimmed milk in some of my fish recipes, but otherwise try and cut down on cow's milk products as much as possible. Switch to organic goat's milk, Soya milk etc – some goat's cheese is fine too, as is a little organic butter now and again. These foods will just enhance the enormous array of wonderfully tasty, nutritious foods that you will be enjoying from now on.

- **Legumes** – I'm personally not a huge fan of legumes (e.g. lentils, pulses, beans and chickpeas etc) as they play havoc with my insides and I think there are generally better, more natural vegetarian food choices available. Nevertheless, I do eat legumes (see recipes) and with careful preparation, they are an excellent source of all the macronutrients and fibre we need in our diet. If you wish to follow a vegetarian or vegan lifestyle, you will certainly need to embrace legumes as a staple of your diet.

- **Nuts and Seeds** – If you have read my book to this point, you will know that I am not the biggest fan of seeds. Nevertheless, I think we should include certain seeds (for example, flaxseed – an excellent vegetarian source of Omega 3) in our diet. Nuts are a good source of healthy macronutrients and would have been a staple of our hunter-gatherer ancestors. Walnuts are a good source of Omega 3 fatty acids and Brazil nuts contain selenium, which is one of our most important micronutrients and often lacking in the modern diet. Sunflower seeds and pumpkin seeds are delicious sprinkled over salads, for instance. Another seed that I love is quinoa, which I eat two or three times a week. So, given my caveat regarding the dangers of eating seeds, which is mostly directed at wheat, please feel free to add some seeds and nuts to your predominantly vegetarian meals as much as you like. You'll find some recipes that include seeds and quinoa later.

Oils and Fats

We looked at oils and liquid fats in some detail earlier, so I don't want to repeat myself too much here. Nevertheless, as this chapter is designed to help you discover the foods you will be eating as the 'new you', I will try and steer you through the oil and fat maze as best I can.

I believe that naturally occurring fats would have been an important part of our ancestral diet and so the 'fats are bad' argument seems not only unnecessarily restrictive, but makes no sense from a biochemical or evolutionary perspective. However, the medical evidence strongly suggests that *excessive* saturated fat in the diet is almost certainly unhealthy as well, so let's see if we can't strike a sensible balance instead.

Omega 6: Omega 3 ratio

First of all, let's get our Omega 6: Omega 3 ratio sorted out. The best way to do this is to include lots of Omega 3 foods in our daily diet (e.g. walnuts, flaxseeds, oily fish etc). I use a teaspoon or so of Udo's Oil on most of my meals, as it tastes delicious and contains a perfect ratio of the Omegas. I also love olive oil and often make olive oil vinaigrette dressing for my salads. As a hopeless grecophile, I am completely obsessed with the wonderful, organic, cold-pressed olive oils from the island of Crete – the best in the world as far as I am concerned. Nevertheless, I am aware that olive oil has a less than perfect Omega 6: Omega 3 ratio (about 15:1, I think) and, as in all oils, it is very energy-rich, providing 9 calories of energy per gram weight. So if, like me, you love olive oil, just remember to go easy on the quantity – just a teaspoon here and there. Also, search out those Cretan oils – they are heavenly!

Saturated fats

Don't get too hung up about saturated fats. Provided we strip the sugar and processed carbs from our diet, we can eat naturally occurring saturated fats in sensible quantities without too much trouble. We certainly don't need to concern ourselves with the natural fats in a portion of healthy, organic meat or poultry for instance, provided we avoid all forms of man-made or trans fats at the same time. I will also let you have a small amount of (organic) butter on your vegetables now and again – just not on toast! Use small amounts of olive oil or Udo's oil on your salads, eat lots of plant foods, throw out the man-made rubbish and don't overly concern yourself with the saturated fats in real, natural foods.

Embrace real foods for easy weight loss

So, there you have it. We have looked at a broad list of foods that we *can* eat as part of our new diet. Please don't dwell on the foods missing from this list – just be prepared to change, change how you view food, change how you buy and prepare food and, most of all, think how *you* will change, in both body shape and health, when you embrace these new wonderful foods. It is now time to turn back the clock and see if we can learn some tips and tricks from our wise elders about how to prepare our meals and otherwise make ends meet.

12

Grandma knew best!

I want to introduce you to a way of buying and preparing real foods based on the tried and tested techniques of our grandparents' generation. This may seem an odd idea at first, but as you will see, there is a lot we can learn from our elders in terms of buying and preparing food, and making ends meet. I will also give you some ideas how to stock the fridge and larder with healthy staples and look at some tips and tricks for planning your shopping and meal preparation. I will cover recipes in more detail at the end of the book. For now, however, we will have a quick look at some of 'Grandma's' cooking ideas, all of which should help you on your way as you prepare for the diet plans to come.

My remarkable grandmother

My grandmother grew up in a poor family around the time of the First World War and so had to learn to make ends meet at a young age. Food was expensive and always in short supply, particularly during post-WW2 rationing. Nevertheless, she managed to feed her entire family remarkably well during those difficult years; above all, food was cherished and treated with respect. This is a far cry from our modern world where food is everywhere we look, whether in petrol stations, railway stations, in supermarkets or available online 24/7.

It was rare to see an obese person in the UK before the 1960s, as in those days few people could afford to overeat. Most meals were eaten at home as eating out was expensive and normally reserved for special occasions. Generally speaking, food was hard to come by and expensive in real terms, so had to be made to 'go a long way'. Meat was particularly expensive meaning certain meals, such as the Sunday roast, were a once–a-week family treat. Leftovers were used to make healthy and delicious meals, often through to midweek. Home cooking, preserving and 'making do' was the order of the day. Many families grew their own fruit and vegetables in the garden.

This was the reality of our grandparents' or great grandparents' generation. People mostly walked or cycled to work, as cars were an expensive luxury beyond the means of most. Apart from popping down to the local 'chippie' for a weekly treat of fish and chips, the idea of ordering a takeaway or buying food at the garage or railway station to eat (in public!) would have been unthinkable. Indeed, many of these wise old ladies would not recognise much of the food we eat today *as* food. They would certainly be appalled at the breakdown in the social structure of mealtimes and the casual, wasteful way we treat food today.

How can Grandma help us today?

We can all learn a great deal from Grandma about how to buy, prepare and eat our food. Many of us have lost sight of the way food used to be prepared and eaten 'back in the day', often in much harder times than now and with effectively less money than we have at our disposal. However, if we can reconnect with these techniques, we will find it much easier to re-establish a healthy relationship with food. Life was hard in pre-War Britain, but how my grandmother's generation coped in terms of 'making ends meet' during those extraordinary times should be an example to us all.

Nowadays, we have a wonderful selection of produce available to us all year round in the shops and supermarkets, which, in real terms, are cheaper than they have ever been. However, many of us have allowed our comfortable, modern life to seduce us into lazy and disorganised eating. Casual meals 'on the go' and takeaways have replaced proper meals made from home-cooked, real food. No, Grandma probably didn't hold down a full-time job, but she almost certainly had less money to spend on food than we do and she certainly didn't have a fully stocked supermarket on her doorstep with amazing produce from all around the World!

Grandma's food tips and tricks

Let's start putting things back together again by using some of the shopping and cooking techniques of these 'wise old ladies'. This should help us return to a structured way of eating, where we eat the right *types* of food at the right *times* of day (i.e. eating properly, in harmony with our evolutionary design, and not grazing all day long on processed foods). If we follow the example of this formidable generation, we can learn to organise ourselves effectively and plan *what* we are going to eat and *when* we are going to do our food shopping. This will help us break the habit of saying "I haven't got any food in the house, I'll get a takeaway". Instead, we can structure a new way of eating around healthy, home-cooked food, just like dear old Grandma.

Many of us are overweight precisely because we do not plan ahead, but instead grab something on the way home from work. However, if we do a bit of planning, we can get the majority of our week's shopping and meal plans worked out over the weekend when most of us have time to sit down for a few minutes and take charge of our lives. With practice, this will become second nature. So, by returning to planning and preparing meals of real foods, eaten at appropriate times of the day, we can avoid the slippery slope of the fast food culture, with its ubiquitous availability and foods containing processed carbohydrate, sugar, trans fats and too many calories.

Eat at the table?

It's entirely up to you of course, but I think it would be great if we could all return to eating more formally at the table. Even if you are on your own, try and reconnect with more structured eating – set yourself a place, get your favourite book and make yourself a proper meal to enjoy at the table. Otherwise, try to return to more traditional mealtimes (e.g. Sunday lunch with the family or making more of an event of the evening meal with your partner, rather than eating off your lap in front of the TV!)

Let's now look at a few possible meal plans based on Grandma's common-sense approach, but updated with foods available to us in the modern World:

A week of meals prepared according to 'Grandma' theory!

(Recipes at the end of the book)

- **Sunday** – Why not have a traditional Sunday lunch with the family? A typical roast might be a joint of meat, usually beef, pork or lamb, but as we are trying to get away from red meat, we'll have a roast chicken instead. All the main supermarkets offer free-range birds these days at reasonable prices, but I urge you to seek out an organic chicken from a reputable local supplier (butcher/farmer etc) if you can. This may cost a bit more, but remember that this quality chicken will form the basis of at least two further meals, so you are saving money in real terms anyway. Roast in the oven, as per my recipe, and add lots of vegetables and salad for a tasty, delicious meal. Fancy a glass of wine? That's up to you, but why not? Enjoy!

- **Monday** – Plenty of leftover chicken for today (if you have a big family, you might have to roast two birds on Sunday), plus the chicken carcass itself and some of the unused vegetables. Off to work on Monday? Take some cold chicken with you, perhaps. Otherwise, you can enjoy a cold chicken salad on Monday evening, plus the rest of the vegetables. This will probably cost you less than a pound – think like Grandma! Keep the chicken carcass covered in the fridge.

- **Tuesday** – Use the chicken carcass as the basis for a stock, throw in some of the remaining vegetables (perhaps add some leeks and turnips) and some red lentils from the store cupboard for a wonderful soup on Tuesday evening. Have some fresh fruit for dessert. Cost? About a pound.

- **Wednesday** – We'll have a mushroom omelette and salad tonight (see recipe section for how to cook the perfect Omelette). Buy six free-range eggs and use three for the omelettte and have the rest for breakfast during the remainder of the week. A pack of organic mushrooms and a bag of salad, and dinner is sorted for a couple of quid. Cooking time is less than ten minutes.

- **Thursday** – How about a vegetable curry? It is too complicated to list the cost of all ingredients (see recipe section), but budget for less than £10 in total. I will allow you to have a small portion of organic brown basmati rice today as a treat.

- **Friday** – Finish off the curry. Perhaps with another salad and yoghurt?

- **Saturday** – Try a big salad with some tinned tuna. Not expensive but delicious, trust me. How about a meal out at the nice French bistro down the road? I would have a Salade Niçoise and a glass of Sancerre. Total cost? No more than a big takeaway and a six pack of beer!

So, that is a sample week, using Grandma principles and in line with the ideas from this book. I know times are hard and I know that junk food is depressingly cheap, but you can eat really healthy, tasty food for not a lot of money. All that is required is a bit of planning and organisation. Please think of yourself *first* – it's not much to ask.

Each of these meals is naturally low in calories (if you go easy on the butter in the chicken and watch the wine consumption) and contain foods that are either very low on the Glycaemic Index or simply don't register on it at all. There is also a distinct lack of sugar in this diet. Each of these meals would take time to digest and hence have only a slow and minimal effect on our insulin levels, too. Result? Lots of healthy nutrients, plentiful portions, no hunger and steady, permanent weight loss.

What's in the pantry?

We've all seen the TV show where the expert goes into someone's house and proceeds to berate them about the contents of their food cupboards and fridge? Well, we are going to be a bit more grown up, so here I have listed some groceries and provisions that I would like you to buy to get you underway with the programme. None of this will cost too much and, of course, these food staples don't need to be bought in one go. You will be eating mostly fresh, real food, so most of this list comprises condiments, designed to enhance the flavour and taste of your natural, real food meals. Consequently, they will last a long time, which in effect makes them cheap. You can add your own ideas, of course, but here are just some of my suggestions for your store cupboard:

- Extra Virgin Olive oil (from the island of Crete).
- Dijon mustard (the smooth, yellow stuff – for my vinaigrette dressing).
- Various curry spices –cumin, cardamom, fenugreek and

coriander etc, as well as some commercial curry powder. Try and buy from an Asian grocer (it's cheaper), as and when you need it. Keep spices in sealed jars for freshness.
- White wine vinegar.
- Udo's oil (health food shops or online).
- Various seeds (e.g. pumpkin, sunflower and flaxseed/linseed) to sprinkle on salads.
- Himalayan salt and black pepper (i.e. pepper cloves in a grinder).
- Organic vegetable stock powder
- Dried (or tinned) organic lentils and chickpeas.
- Rapeseed oil.
- Organic brown basmati rice (for an occasional treat).
- Tinned fish – tuna, mackerel and sardines (try and buy tinned fish in spring water and make sure it is both dolphin-friendly and MSC approved).
- Quinoa (a true 'wonder' food and the sacred food of the Incas).
- Some Asian food staples (e.g. rice wine, sesame oil, soy sauce etc).

We are just trying to return to a way of eating that puts real food at the centre of each and every meal. By doing a bit of planning, we can soon learn to make delicious, satisfying meals for all the family. By thinking like Grandma, not only can we re-establish a healthy relationship with food, we can lose weight, kick the junk food habit and spend *less* money on food than we did before. It's another win-win situation!

Real food deserves our respect

Our grandparents' generation seems to have shown more respect for food than we do today, which makes sense when you think how relatively poor they were and how difficult it was to get hold of high-quality foods in post-War Britain. Today, we seem to treat eating as a tedious inconvenience that has to be fitted in and around the mad rush of our chaotic working lives and our equally chaotic social lives. And, as we now know, this approach to food is a major factor in the current obesity epidemic. So, let's rewind and get back to putting real food at the centre of our lives, just like Grandma did. It's time to get back to living like Grandma, at least in terms of how we buy and prepare food (knitting optional!).

13

Seven weeks to change your life: The Back to Basics Diet

It is now time to say farewell to your old sedentary life of processed, sugary foods and embrace a healthy, real food diet instead. It is also high time that you thought about you for a change by putting yourself first every day.

What follows is a seven-week programme designed to ease you into a new, healthy way of life. Instead of trying to lose weight by following one fad diet after another, the Back to Basics programme will give you a diet and lifestyle template, which you can follow step-by-step as you begin to change your life for the better. This is not some sort of quick fix; instead, you will be asked to make some fundamental changes to your diet and given tips for how to go about getting active everyday.

By following the programme closely over the seven weeks, you will learn how to change your shopping and cooking habits and will discover the joy of just 'getting outside' by walking everyday. Once you have got the hang of this initial phase, you can start to play around with recipes, food ideas and types of daily activity to suit your own lifestyle. This way, the Back to Basics programme becomes a template to help you make the right food and activity choices for the rest of your life.

Make a contract with me

I now want you to enter into a contract with me. From your side, I want you to get organised, do some planning in preparation for the 'new you' and employ a modicum of willpower to help you change from your old habits to the new habits in the Back to Basics programme. For my part, I have laid out some detailed diet and lifestyle plans that will help you get underway with the necessary changes you need to make to lose weight, get fit and active, and generally feel good about yourself once again. So, let's shake hands and agree to work together to make sure you get the maximum benefit from the programme.

Nobody will nag you, laugh at you, scold you or poke fun at you here. All you have to do is pick *one* of the two programmes, read through it a couple of times, get organised with your shopping and meal preparation, and follow it day-by-day. Then, watch the pounds fall away as you rediscover the joy of simply being alive.

Seven weeks to change your life

I want to make sure you take your time to adjust to your new, healthy way of life, so I suggest you take things one day at a time. There are seven days in a week – so in week one, I want you to follow the Back to Basics programme to the letter on *one* day that week. In week two, I want you to follow the programme for *two* days a week and so on. After seven weeks, you will have completed the transition from your 'bad', old lifestyle to the Back to Basics programme in nice, easy stages. This simple seven-week programme is summarised here:

The Back to Basics Seven-Week Diet programme

Weeks	Follow the Back to Basics programme on:
Week One	One day
Week Two	Two days
Week Three	Three days
Week Four	Four days
Week Five	Five days
Week Six	Six days
Week Seven	All week!

Once you have reached week seven, just stick with it. I have included a few recipes at the end of the book to help you on your way, but from week eight onwards, I want *you* to take responsibility for *your* life by researching new recipes and new ways to be active everyday. If you ever start to 'wobble' or want someone else to do the thinking for you for a while, come back to the programme and follow it closely until you are happy to go solo once more. Just follow your chosen plan and you will be fine.

However you spin it, the Back to Basics programme will give you lots of nutrients and will help you eat fewer calories than you burn up through your daily activity. All the while, you will be keeping your insulin levels under control, with all the associated benefits we have discussed. The Back to Basics programme is simple, straightforward, easy to follow and will change your life for the better and forever.

The Back to Basics Diet Plans

You can choose one of *two* plans on the Back to Basics programme. Most of you should choose the basic programme unless you are injured or infirm, in which case you should start with the modified programme – aimed at those of you who are unable to exercise due to injury or disability. Each plan combines healthy meal choices, alteration to meal timings and daily activity into one, holistic system that you can follow for the rest of your life. No tricks, no gimmicks, just eating in accordance with your evolutionary design.

Each plan has been designed around the main principles of this book (i.e. the use of intermittent fasting to minimise the time spent insulinated, making best use of low insulin levels to access fat reserves, and daily activity to really burn off the fat once and for all). Each plan will also encourage positive thinking to help you on your way. Regardless of which one you choose, your Back to Basics diet plan will contain the following types and quantities of foods:

Types of food:

- Real, natural foods that provide *high* levels of nutrients for *low* amounts of calories. Your meals will be based around fruit, salads and vegetables – all of which are relatively energy poor (i.e. *low* in calories, but nutrient-rich; full of phytochemicals, vitamins, anti-oxidants, proteins and healthy fats that are essential for health). This sort of food takes a while to digest, so by filling up on low-calorie, nutrient-rich plant food, we simply won't be able to eat too many calories in any given time period. If we then add sensible portions of poultry, fish, vegetable protein, and healthy fats – all eaten at the appropriate times of the day – we pretty much arrive at our perfect diet. This is very different to the bad 'old diet' of our past and the highly processed, high-calorie, low-nutrient foods that made us fat.

- 80%-90% of each meal should comprise high-quality (preferably organic) vegetables and fruit. Green vegetables and wild fruits (e.g. berries) are the panacea to good health.

- The remainder of your diet (10-20%) should be high-quality protein from vegetables, organic fish, organic poultry, eggs, nuts and healthy fats.

- If you must eat red meat, eat it rarely and make sure it is organic or wild game (venison etc). Best to avoid altogether, I'm afraid.

- Use *organic olive oil* or a *balanced Omega 6: Omega 3* oil, such as Udo's Oil, as your primary fat source – add some flaxseed to your meals, too.

- The odd glass of wine is perfectly OK. If you are really struggling, an occasional baked potato, *single* piece of wholemeal bread or small portion of brown rice is fine once in a while.

Quantities of food:

- I haven't mentioned portion size that much so far, as I think it is much more important to emphasise the types of food we should eat, rather than to fixate on portion control. Nevertheless, I think sensible portion control just means eating until we are pleasantly replete, *not* completely stuffed. By concentrating on the types of food in our meals, the calories will largely take care of themselves. However, if you want a bit more guidance, try eating no more food at each meal than you could hold in two-cupped hands – as recommended by Gudrun Jonsson in her famous book, *The Gut Reaction*.

Timings of meals and snacks

So, *when* are we going to eat? We are going to eat to maximise the low insulin phases of the day (i.e. as late as possible in the morning, after we have taken our morning activity and early in the evening, again after another bout of activity). This way, we spend as much time as possible in the fat-burning zone, when we are primed to burn fat, not store it. So, try and eat your first meal of the day as late in the morning as possible. At the very least, make sure you do some activity before eating breakfast.

Eventually, I would like you to try and squeeze your eating into a small segment of the day (e.g. brunch/early lunch around midday, afternoon snack and early evening meal). Whatever you do, don't graze. Grazing just means we keep eating calories all day long *and* keep our insulin levels permanently elevated. That's a 'lose-lose' scenario. If you do get hungry, have another snack of fruit or raw vegetables, or in extremis, another 'two-cupped hands' meal. Stick to the rules of the game and you shouldn't ever get hungry. You will be eating plenty of food at similar times each day, which will help your system settle down and relieve those dreaded hunger pangs.

Treats

I am not a big fan of treats – I think the idea that we can get away with a bit of 'naughty' food now and again is misguided and in truth a failure to completely commit to a healthy diet and lifestyle. There are plenty of treats available from real food, without resorting to eating rubbish once again. Sweet tooth? Eat some fruit or have some honey. Still got a sweet craving? Don't worry; the cravings won't last long. Your body is changing from a sugar-addicted, low-nutrient version of 'you' to a new, healthy, high-nutrient version, so hang in there because the cravings will soon pass.

Here's a tip, which works for alcohol and tobacco cravings too – drink a glass of water and go out for a walk. Get addicted to activity instead. Got addictions to booze, drugs or tobacco? Go and get help; there is plenty of it out there. Want to improve your self-esteem in one fell swoop? Stub out that cigarette and get off the booze – you will feel much better about yourself, trust me.

Activity

Take things easy at first – start by walking every day and see how you go. If you are very heavy and/or very unfit, have a chat with your doctor before you start. Save up and buy yourself a heart rate monitor and some trainers because it will make all the difference. Go outside and get active first thing in the morning (make it part of your journey to work, for instance) and try and go for a walk again before you sit down to your evening meal. Don't worry about what other people think – just get out of that front door. Here are some activity suggestions:

- Get up and go out for a walk.
- Walk or cycle to work.
- Walk the kids to school and back home again in the afternoon.
- Cycle with the kids to school.
- Get a dog – no excuses for not walking then!
- Go swimming.
- Join a gym if you wish, but not necessary in the early stages.
- Dance round the house to your iPod.
- Use a TV fitness programme.
- Take up a sport.
- Take up a martial art.
- Dig the garden.

I suggest you try walking at first and then just get on with it. Remember, this is daily activity, so make it part of your life. Very soon, you won't believe how you could have lived for so long without being active.

Are you scared of falling off the wagon?

The diet and lifestyle changes in the Back to Basics diet may seem daunting at first, but they are actually very straightforward and will soon become second nature once you have completed the initial seven-week programme. Nevertheless, there are bound to be a few hiccups along the way, so please don't worry too much if you have the occasional wobble. Just pick yourself up and carry on with the programme – you'll get there in the end. Be mindful and remember why you are trying to change. It is time to look after *you* and address your weight, your health and your happiness at last. Everything has to come second to that, just for a while.

Mindful action

One of the hardest things for us to do in life is to be selfish and think about ourselves *first*. None of us are naturally selfish and we have spent a lifetime looking after our partners, our children and our friends before thinking about *our* needs at all. If we are not mindful of our own needs, it is easy to be lulled into temptation when our minds are elsewhere, thinking about all the other people who depend on us. So, to help you stay focused in the face of temptation, here is a tip I picked up from a completely different part of my life (scuba diving, actually) that works brilliantly in the context of sticking to changes in your diet. The next time you are caught off-guard and tempted by a sandwich, a piece of toast or a cream bun, try this:

'STOP, BREATHE, THINK, ACT!'

This only takes a second: before you instinctively order that sandwich or pick up a packet of biscuits at the petrol station, just *stop* for a moment. Take a deep *breath*, *think* about what you are doing and then *turn away* – it's that easy. It's all about putting you *first*. Just stop, breathe, think and act!

Choosing your Back to Basics Diet Plan

What follows is a choice of diet plan and which plan you choose depends entirely on your personal circumstances. Each plan provides a suggested structure for the next few weeks of your life and is designed to help you on your way to a healthy weight. After the initial seven-week phase, feel free to stick with your particular plan for as long as you like. When you are ready, you can change over to the 'Maintenance Programme', a slightly modified version of the Back to Basics diet, which will allow you to continue eating healthily for the rest of your life. Have a look at each plan in turn and choose *one* to get you started. Most of you should stick with the 'Basic' plan, but whichever plan you choose, you will be find a weeks' worth of meals and detailed advice as to how to structure your day around your new, healthy eating regime.

Nevertheless, you must be prepared to change. You must accept that to lose weight, you need to change *what* you eat, *when* you eat and your whole attitude to exercise. Take a deep breath and prepare to begin your new life. Are you ready? Let's get to it!

14

The Back to Basics Diet Plans

Welcome to the Back to Basics diet and lifestyle plans. Each plan is specifically designed to provide you with a framework of meals and daily activity around which you can structure each and every day for the rest of your life. This is *not* a quick fix solution, but a programme designed to help you make significant changes to your diet and lifestyle to ensure you beat the obesity 'ogre', once and for all.

Don't lose sight of why you need to lose weight

People who love you and care about you have been desperate for you to lose weight for years, simply because they *do* love you and want you to be healthy and around for a while longer yet. Meanwhile, you and I have been told to 'eat less and move more' or 'cut down' or 'watch our portion size' or 'eat healthily' or 'just take more exercise' until we are blue in the face. So far, these well-meaning suggestions haven't been much use, have they? Faced with this barrage of contradictory advice, we have stumbled from one diet to another, taking 'one step forward and two steps back', before eventually losing heart and reverting to our self-imposed misery and another packet of biscuits. Remember, I speak from experience!

Let's now put all that in the past. If you want, you could now just change your diet to one comprising real, unprocessed food, start taking daily activity and leave it at that. I pretty much guarantee that over time, your weight would come down and you would be a much, healthier, happier person all round. However, we can do better. By following one of the Back to Basics diet plans, you will be able to maximise your ability to lose weight *and* make sure you keep that weight off in the future. By eating real, unprocessed foods at set times, you will naturally reduce your calorie intake and allow your insulin levels to stabilise at a lower level for most of the day. And by taking activity when you are *best* able to burn your fat (i.e. when your insulin levels are low), you will fit the final piece into the weight-loss jigsaw and markedly improve your chances of lifelong, permanent weight loss. You will also feel full for most of the day, so will be able to break the habit of grazing on processed foods and snacks all day long because you will not be hungry.

It's time to fall in love with real food again

Follow your chosen diet programme step-by-step and you will have no choice but to plan your meals and food shopping ahead of time (e.g. prepare packed lunches for work) and build daily activity into your life. Above all, your Back to Basics diet plan is a way for you to re-establish a healthy relationship with food; the days of grabbing some cheap junk food at the first sign of sugar-induced hunger are over. Just follow your chosen plan, followed by the subsequent 'Maintenance Programme' and you will eat fewer calories than you burn up through your daily activity and give your body more nutrients than it has probably ever had before. All the while, you will be losing weight steadily, day-by-day, as you begin your journey to the new 'you'.

The rules of the game

It will probably help you to stay on the straight and narrow if you keep a few 'rules of the game' in mind in the weeks and months ahead. The beauty of the Back to Basics programme is that it doesn't rely on fads or weird ingredients or recipes that only a Michelin-starred chef could understand. Just keep the following rules in mind when shopping, preparing meals at home or eating out because they will help you make the *correct* choices – at least until such choices become second nature:

- **Only eat real foods** – fruit, salads, vegetables, fish, organic poultry, fresh eggs, nuts and organic meats.

- **Avoid all forms of processed foods** – takeaways, sandwiches, ready meals, fast foods, breads, cakes, pastries, sugary snacks, savoury snacks, beer and sodas

- Think before reaching for a sandwich or cake *out of habit* – stop, breathe, think and act.

- **Eating out is easy** – choose your protein (ideally fish, chicken or vegetarian) and add lots of vegetables and salad. Say 'no thank you' to starters, puddings, bread rolls, chips and pints of beer. Enjoy your meal, have a glass of wine if you wish and remain safe in the knowledge that you are losing weight and still on your path to health and happiness.

- **Eat loads of green things** – salads, vegetables and fruit. Eat these foods until you are pleasantly full. If you get hungry between meals, eat more green things.

- **Take daily activity** – go for a walk, cycle or swim twice a day. Make sure you are active before eating your first meal of the day and again before your evening meal. That means every day – no exceptions.

- **Try and enjoy life** – treasure the good times, love your partner and your kids, see your friends, go out and socialise (following the rules about eating out). It's an old cliché, but life is not a rehearsal – make the most of every day.

- **Over to you** – losing weight and regaining your health and happiness is in your hands. Make the most of this opportunity and just go for it.

The Back to Basics step-by-step system

To help you get underway with making the changes in your life that will be inevitable as you take your first tentative steps with your chosen plan, I suggest you follow this simple step-by-step guide:

- **Step 1 – Choose a plan.**
- **Step 2 – Get organised.**
- **Step 3 – Identify your addiction triggers.**
- **Step 4 – Go shopping.**
- **Step 5 – Take a deep breath and go for it.**

STEP 1 – Choose a plan

Most of you should choose the 'Basic Plan', as this includes normal levels of daily activity. However, if you are infirm or otherwise unable to exercise, I have included a slightly modified version that puts more emphasis on restricting calories through strict portion control. Nevertheless, you will be encouraged to do whatever you can in terms of getting active each day as well. Whichever plan you choose, move onto the 'Maintenance Programme' when you are ready after the initial seven-week phase.

STEP 2 – Get organised

You will need to get organised before getting underway with

your chosen plan, so take a few minutes to sit down quietly at some point with pen and paper and do a bit of planning. Which day of the week will you start your seven-week initial phase? Which meals/recipes do you want to try? What do you need to buy to stock up your store cupboard? Just give yourself the time to think about these sorts of questions before you rush headlong into the programme.

STEP 3 – Identify your addiction triggers

Many of us who are overweight know full well that we have a soft spot for certain types of food or drink – the 'comforts' we turn to when we are feeling fed up or depressed. What's important is that we own up to this in our own minds; be honest with yourself about your eating habits and lay your cards on the table before going any further. In my case, I turned to savoury snacks in moments of weakness and at my lowest ebb, I drank too much – something I have now addressed successfully. This is not an easy thing for me, or anyone else, to admit; we often feel 'weak' or 'pathetic' and beat ourselves up without really ever addressing the problem itself.

Now is the time to be brutally honest. If you have serious addictions to drugs or alcohol, or have an eating disorder such as bulimia, please go and get help. Talk to your doctor in the first instance and take it from there. Otherwise, just work out what it is that triggers any 'naughty' food behaviour and be aware of it as you begin your diet plan. The Back to Basics programme should keep you on the straight and narrow, but if you feel yourself wobbling for any reason, just stop, breathe, think and act. Got a sweet tooth? Eat some fruit, not a chocolate biscuit. Feeling peckish? Drink a glass of water and walk around the block. If that doesn't work, eat some fruit, nuts, raw vegetables or a piece of protein (e.g. some cold chicken). Just keep your eye on the big picture – it's all about *you*, so hang in there!

STEP 4 – Go shopping

It's time now to stock your fridge and larder with real foods. Follow my suggested list of essentials in chapter eleven and work out where you are going to source the fresh foods for each day of the plan. Visit your local farmers' market and make friends with some of the stallholders. Perhaps join a box scheme and get organic vegetables and fruit delivered to your door. Can you grow your own?

Go to your local supermarket and conduct a recce – what are their fruit and vegetables like? How expensive is it compared to the other supermarket down the road? How much organic produce do they have? Do you want to go shopping every couple of days or would you rather get a home delivery? It is time to put yourself *first*; shopping for real foods like this is central to that process, so take your time and work out a way of food shopping that suits you.

STEP 5 – Take a deep breath and go for it

Are you ready to get started? Have you organised your life, explained what you are doing to your friends and family and stocked the larder with lots of lovely, healthy fresh fruits, salads and vegetables? Do you need to look back over the book to refresh your memory about certain aspects of the theory or are you happy to go for it?

The diet plans follow overleaf – just stick to the rules and remember that this is a seven-week initial programme, as follows:

Weeks	Follow the Back to Basics programme on:
Week One	One day
Week Two	Two days
Week Three	Three days
Week Four	Four days
Week Five	Five days
Week Six	Six days
Week Seven	All week!

So, off you go. I'm sure you will love it and won't look back once you get started. Good luck!

The 'Basic Plan'

- Alarm clock goes off, it's time to get up!

- **It's time to get active** – Get out of bed and go for a walk or otherwise do your morning activity. Build it into your journey to work (walk, cycle etc) if necessary. Walk the kids to school, perhaps.

- **Breakfast** – Have a cup of tea or coffee if you like, but see if you can hold out till later in the morning before eating. If that is simply too difficult, just make sure you wait until *after* your morning activity before eating your breakfast.

- **Brunch/Lunch** – Try and make this the *first meal* of the day. That way, you can maximise your overnight fast before raising your insulin levels again when you eat. If you *do* eat breakfast, do *not* eat again until later in the day (i.e. have a late lunch, not a brunch two hours after breakfast). Remember, we are trying to control our calories *and* let our insulin levels drop back to a resting level as much as possible between meals.

- **Afternoon snack** – Try some fresh fruit or raw vegetables with hummus or a handful of nuts.

- **It's time to be active again** – Do some form of activity (in the late afternoon or early evening) before you eat your dinner. Go for a walk or build it into your day (walk, cycle home from work, play with the kids in the garden/back yard/local park or go to the gym).

- **Evening meal** – Choose *one* from: fish with vegetables/salad, vegetable protein with vegetables/salad or chicken/turkey with vegetables/salad. Add spices and flavours as much as you like. Use olive oil or Udo's Oil in moderation for salad dressing and don't worry too much about fat on meat. Enjoy a glass of wine if you wish (just one), but no pudding. Have some fresh fruit instead. See more meal ideas overleaf and my recipes at the back of the book.

- **Time to relax** – Enjoy some quality time with your partner, family and friends. Read a book, watch a movie, talk about your holiday plans and tell your partner how much you love them. It's time to rediscover happiness in life.

- **Bedtime** – Over to you!

I have listed a few suggested meals for the 'Basic Plan' below. Once you are comfortable eating this way, try and work out your own meal plans and recipes to suit you. I've tried to keep things as simple as possible (I am a man!) and have listed a few ideas that you can try for either brunch or dinner. I have included some recipe ideas at the back of the book. Ideally, try and just eat *two* main meals a day.

Some brunch suggestions

- Fresh fruit.
- Berry fruits (strawberries, raspberries, blueberries etc) and goat's yoghurt.
- Strawberries and champagne (wedding anniversary?).
- Omelette and salad.
- Bacon and mushrooms.
- Bacon and eggs.
- Scrambled eggs and smoked salmon.
- Porridge oats (a bit 'carby', but OK in moderation if you must).
- Bircher muesli (ditto).
- Dave's Kedgeree.
- Smoked haddock and poached egg.
- Kippers.
- Certain cereals are OK (e.g. Nature's Path gluten-free Organic Mesa Sunrise).

Some dinner suggestions

- Salade Niçoise (see recipe suggestion).
- Huge salad plus some chicken, fish or cold meats.
- Vegetable curry (ideally no rice, but you can have a small portion of organic brown basmati rice if you wish).
- Vegetable soup (no bread).
- Healthy chicken and vegetable soup.
- Dave's One-Minute Wonder Salad plus tuna, cold

chicken or roast beef.
- Gilly's Wonderful Asian Fish (or similar recipe).
- Quinoa and salad.
- Steak and salad.
- Pork chops and vegetables.
- Roast chicken plus steamed vegetables.

Off to work? Some ideas for packed brunch and/or lunch:

- Cold chicken plus salad/vegetables.
- Hard-boiled eggs plus salad/vegetables.
- Tomatoes, raw carrots and celery, plus a pot of hummus.
- Berries and yoghurt.
- Crudities.
- Tin of tuna plus salad, raw vegetables and a little mayo?
- Some homemade soup in a flask.

Bring some salad dressing from home (see Dave's Vinaigrette recipe) and buy the following from the canteen, staff restaurant or local shop: salads, vegetables, chicken breast, fish, turkey, ham etc.

Some tips and tricks for the 'Basic Plan'

Remember, try and cook like Grandma – buy a good quality joint/chicken, make it last two or three meals, make stock, make soups and grow your own vegetables. Basically, use any combination of healthy protein (i.e. fish, chicken, turkey, eggs, or vegetable foods like lentils, chickpeas, hummus) with lots of salad and vegetables. Red meat is OK in moderation, but there is some evidence that excessive red meat consumption *might* be carcinogenic, so chicken, fish and vegetable protein is safer. I will allow you some berry fruit for 'afters' (strawberries and cream are great in the summer).

Don't worry too much about calories or portion size. This is not a restriction diet. By eating real, natural food and being reasonably sensible with your portion size (e.g. Gudrun Jonssen's 'two-cupped hands'), the calories will look after themselves. All we are really trying to do is to get rid of the sugar (processed carbs) and go back to eating real food. If you're hungry, have another 'two-cupped hands' snack.

Once you are comfortable with the Back to Basics diet, have a go at creating your own meals to suit *you*. Keep it simple – combine real, organic protein with salad/vegetables. There is no need for complex or highfalutin recipes here. Try having my 'One-Minute Wonder Salad' at each meal, either as a main course or as a side dish. Make your own version and take it to work, eat it for supper or have it for breakfast. Remember, you must eat a predominantly vegetarian diet.

Feel free to use your own recipes and meal ideas as you wish. Just stick to the principles:

- **Get up.**
- **Activity.**

- **Brunch/lunch.**
- **Afternoon snack.**
- **Activity.**
- **Dinner.**

Here is a sample week (from week seven onwards) on the 'Basic Plan':

Remember – eat *plenty* of food at each meal

	Am activity	Brunch	Snack	Pm activity	Dinner
Monday	Walk, cycle, swim etc	Cold chicken, salad/vegetables	Fresh fruit	Walk, cycle, swim etc	My 'One Minute Wonder' salad
Tuesday	"	Tuna salad	Nuts and vegetables	"	Homemade soup
Wednesday	"	Omelette and salad	Fresh fruit	"	Smoked haddock and vegetables
Thursday	"	Vegetable curry	Fresh fruit	"	Quinoa and salad
Friday	"	Salmon salad	Nuts and vegetables	"	Dave's dall and vegetables
Saturday	"	Bacon and mushrooms	Crudities and hummus	"	Salade Niçoise
Sunday	"	Sunday roast	Fresh fruit	"	Cold cuts and salad

The modified 'Basic Plan'

A very infirm friend of mine asked me if I could tweak the Back to Basics diet for those who are unable to take *any* activity, due to injury, illness or disability. Here, then, is a slightly modified version of the 'Basic Plan', designed to help you still lose weight effectively even if you are unable to take any activity at all.

What follows here is very similar to the 'Basic Plan' but with more emphasis on calorie control. Unfortunately, you are going to have to be *much* more aware of your calorie consumption, compared to those of us who have no excuse but to take daily activity. You can, if you want, work out your own BMI (see Appendix 1) and then apply strict calorie counting at each meal. However, that's a complete pain, so instead I recommend you follow the 'Basic Plan' but use *rigorous* portion control at each meal (as per the 'two-cupped hands').

Most of us who are obese, regardless of our current ability to be active or not, have got that way through a lifetime's overconsumption of processed foods and sugar. Even if you are unable to take any activity but follow my advice to the letter, you will still be dramatically reducing your calorie consumption compared to your 'bad old diet' anyway. Nevertheless, to ensure that you really make inroads into your excess weight, you must be *very* strict about portion size and number of snacks. You have very little leeway on your calorie intake if we are to get that weight moving. So, stick to *two* meals per day (which must be no larger than 'two cupped' hands) and *one* mid-afternoon snack. Don't worry too much – the wonderful, tasty, natural food you will eat from now on, albeit in fairly concise portions, will still fill you up, reduce your hunger pangs, make you lose weight and, above all, make you feel better about yourself than perhaps you have ever done before.

Some tips and tricks for the modified 'Basic Plan'

My advice here is much the same as the 'Basic Plan'. Try and cook like Grandma – buy a good quality joint/chicken, make it last two or three meals, make stock, make soups and grow your own veg. Just use any combination of healthy protein, whether fish, chicken, turkey, eggs, cheese, or vegetable foods like lentils, chickpeas, hummus with lots of salad and vegetables. Red meat is OK in moderation, but there is some evidence that excessive consumption *might* be carcinogenic, so chicken, fish and vegetable protein is safer. I will allow you some berry fruit for 'afters' (strawberries and cream are great in summer). Just concentrate on portion control.

We are still just trying to get rid of the sugar (processed carbs) and go back to eating *real* food. So, if you get really hungry, have another 'two-cupped hands' snack.

Once you are comfortable with the Back to Basics diet, have a go at creating your own meals to suit *you*. Keep it simple – combine real, organic protein with salad/vegetables; there is no need for complex or highfalutin recipes here. Try having my 'One-Minute Wonder Salad' at each meal, either as a main course or as a side dish. Make your own version and take it to work, eat it for supper or have it for breakfast. Remember, we just need to eat a *predominantly* vegetarian diet.

Here's your plan:

- Alarm clock goes off, it's time to get up.

- Try and do *some* sort of activity now. This is entirely up to you, but there is often something you can do to get the heartbeat raised a bit. When my mother had a hip replacement and couldn't walk for a few weeks, she sat in a chair and did some stretches and arm swinging to her favourite music. So, try and do some sort of activity now if you can, before you eat breakfast. *Any* activity that will make you huff and puff a bit will help you burn some calories and so make it easier for you to start getting that weight moving. You will also help improve your fitness and make you feel better about yourself, too. See what you can do and just go for it.

- **Breakfast** – Have a cup of tea or coffee if you want, but see if you can hold out until later in the morning before eating. I'm not anti-breakfast as such, so if that is simply too difficult, please enjoy a healthy breakfast now. Just make sure you eat *after* your morning activity.

- **Brunch/lunch –** Try and make this the *first* meal of the day. That way, you can maximise your overnight fast before raising your insulin levels again when you eat. If you *do* eat breakfast, do *not* eat again until later in the day (have a late lunch, not a brunch two hours after breakfast). Remember, we are trying to control our calories *and* let our insulin levels drop back to a resting level as much as possible between meals. Here though, you have to be very careful about portion size. Remember, 'two cupped hands' – no more.

- **Afternoon snack –** Try some fresh fruit or raw vegetables with hummus or a handful of nuts.

- **It's time for activity again –** Sometime in the late afternoon or early evening, try and do *some* form of activity before dinner. Again, this depends entirely on your personal circumstances, but have a think about it and see if you can work out some way you can burn a few calories now.

- **Evening meal –** Choose *one* from: fish with vegetables/salad, vegetable protein with vegetables/salad or chicken/turkey with vegetables/salad. (Add spices and flavours as much as you like. Use olive oil or Udo's Oil in moderation for salad dressing and don't worry too much about fat on meat. Enjoy a glass of wine if you wish (just one), but no pudding. Have some fresh fruit instead. Remember: strict portion control. 'Two-cupped hands' only! See more meal ideas overleaf and my recipes at the back of the book.

- **Time to relax** – Enjoy some quality time with your partner, family or friends. Read a book, watch a movie, talk about your holiday plans and tell your partner how much you love them. It's time to rediscover happiness in life.

- **Bedtime** – Over to you!

Use the same meal/recipe ideas from the 'Basic Plan' but, as always, feel free to use your own recipes and meal ideas as you wish. Just stick to the 'rules of the game' and really focus on portion control:

- **Get up.**
- **Activity.**
- **Brunch/lunch.**
- **Afternoon snack.**
- **Activity.**
- **Dinner.**

Here is a sample week (from week seven onwards) on the modified 'Basic Plan'. Remember that portion control is key to your success – 'two-cupped hands'.

	Am activity	Brunch	Snack	Pm activity	Dinner
Monday	Walk, cycle, swim etc	Cold chicken, salad/vegetables	Fresh fruit	Walk, cycle, swim etc	My 'One Minute Wonder' salad
Tuesday	"	Tuna salad	Nuts and vegetables	"	Homemade soup
Wednesday	"	Omelette and salad	Fresh fruit	"	Smoked haddock and vegetables
Thursday	"	Vegetable curry	Fresh fruit	"	Quinoa and salad
Friday	"	Salmon salad	Nuts and vegetables	"	Dave's dall and vegetables

The Back to Basics 'Maintenance Programme'

Stick to the rules of the game

The Back to Basics programme is designed as a *framework* around which you can plan your daily eating and activity for the rest of your life. Therefore, I suggest you move onto what I call the 'Maintenance Plan' after the initial seven-week transition phase. There is no great mystery about this – it is simply a slightly more relaxed version of the 'Basic Plan'.

The 'Basic Plan' is obviously designed for weight loss, but it also functions as a template for you to follow for the rest of your life. So, what do we need to alter to make the 'Basic Plan' suitable as a lifelong template for weight management and healthy living? Well, we know we need to take daily activity, so the morning activity session (before we eat anything) stays put. I still suggest you stick to eating a late brunch or an early lunch in preference to breakfast, but if your weight is stable, feel free to have something to eat straight after your morning activity if you so wish. Similarly, the afternoon activity session before dinner also stays, so no real change there. You can have your afternoon snack as normal.

So, what else needs to change? Not much, really. The beauty of the 'Basic Plan' is that it not only helps us lose weight and change to eating in accordance with our design as healthy humans, it also serves as our daily guide through life as well. Two meals per day of real, natural, unprocessed food (predominantly vegetarian), a fresh fruit or vegetable snack, plus daily activity is all we need to remain healthy and happy for the rest of our lives. It's as simple as that!

You will probably be able to eat larger portions at each sitting if you wish. In this case, keep an eye on your weight and if it starts to creep up, go back to 'two-cupped hands' and you will soon lose any extra pounds. You can make any combinations of foods you want at each meal too, provided you stick to the rules. Just remember, forget about treats (i.e. cakes, pastries, takeaways and junk food) – that's all in the past. You have made a huge change to your life so don't throw that away now, after all the good work you have done. Feel free to experiment and try lots of healthy new recipes; however, please don't worry if you haven't cooked much before because you don't need to be a gourmet chef to follow these diet plans. Try my recipes to start with (particularly my 'One-Minute Wonder Salad' and my super-quick and easy brunches) and see how you get on. After that, you can follow any recipe you like – just remember to avoid processed food.

15

Final thoughts

I hope you have enjoyed reading this book and I sincerely hope my advice will help you regain control of your weight *and* boost your health and happiness. I am delighted that many people are now following the programme and reporting great success along the way (I talk about this and many other aspects of the programme on my blog at www.thebacktobasicsdiet.com). Nevertheless, this book isn't about me – it's about you. Quite deliberately, I have put a lot of emphasis on you learning to put yourself first in life. Our obesity problems stem not only from a bad diet, but also from a lack of care and attention to how we eat and otherwise live our lives. Most of us know intuitively that we shouldn't be eating much of the food we eat, even if we don't quite know why. However, what and when we eat is usually one of the last decisions we make each day, not the first. So from now on, put that right by following my plan and put yourself *first* in your list of priorities.

I just want to finish on this final point. You are a unique, wonderful human being who deserves to be healthy and happy in life. I know the misery that can ensue once we lose control of our eating and drinking and start to pile on the pounds. If nothing else: by taking steps to lose weight and return to full health, your own self-confidence and self-esteem will receive a huge boost. That, all by itself, is a cause for celebration.

However, there is more. Even if you are currently at a low ebb, just realise that you are loved – loved by partners, children, parents and close friends, probably more than you can imagine. I recently lost a very dear friend to cancer. She was fifty-seven-years-old and rather famous in her own right. At her funeral, mourners stood ten deep outside the crematorium because it was full. Five hundred people attended her memorial service. Her husband, so obviously devastated himself, remarked that she would *never* have believed how many people had come to see her off. That was because many, many people loved her, far more than she would have ever realised when she was alive. And that goes for you, too.

So, while you are working away at your new diet plan, remember that there is more to life than food. Enjoy each and every day. Look around at the people you love and remember that they love you, too. Spend time with them, laugh with them and share meals together – real food meals only, please! Enjoy a glass of wine or two together and remember that life is for living. Cherish each and every day you are alive and remember that by putting yourself first, you are *not* being selfish but ensuring that you can be surrounded by people who love you for as long as possible and vice versa.

Many thanks for reading the book.

All the best
David

16

Recipes

I have included some of my favourite recipes here to help you
on your way with the Back to Basics diet. Provided you continue
to play by the rules, you are free to work out your own delicious,
healthy meal ideas as you progress with the plan. (For further
recipe ideas, see my blog at www.thebacktobasicsdiet.com). Just
remember to have lots of vegetables and salad with each of these
meal ideas.

I though it might be useful if I grouped the recipe ideas
into two groups: 'Super-quick and Easy Brunches' and
'Quick and Easy Dinners'. Obviously, this is not a rigid list,
but is just intended to give you a basic guide to help you
decide which meals to prepare and when, depending on
your own lifestyle.

Super-quick and Easy Brunches:

- Astronaut's breakfast.
- Mushroom omelette.
- Kippers.
- Scrambled eggs and bacon.
- Scrambled eggs and smoked salmon.

- Smoked haddock and poached egg.
- Dave's Kedgeree.
- Dave's One-Minute Wonder Salad (recipe in 'Dinners' section).

Quick and Easy Dinners

- Dave's Roast Chicken.
- Healthy chicken and vegetable soup.
- Dave's Veggie Curry.
- Dave's One-Minute Wonder Salad.
- Gilly's Wonderful Asian Fish.
- Dave's Quinoa Salad.
- Dave's Tarka Dall.
- Salade Niçoise.

Super-quick and Easy Brunches

Astronaut's breakfast

As eaten by NASA astronauts in the Apollo era – ideal for a special weekend treat.
Ingredients:
- An organic beef steak (fillet or sirloin).
- A knob of organic butter.
- Salt and pepper.
- One or two fresh organic eggs.
- Some organic butter.

- Rapeseed oil.
- White wine vinegar.

Take a small organic piece of beef fillet steak or sirloin steak and season with salt and pepper. Heat a teaspoon of oil in a frying pan and turn up the heat. Add a knob of organic butter. When it has stopped foaming, place the steak in the pan. Cook a couple of minutes on each side or otherwise to taste. Meanwhile, boil some water in a saucepan. Add a teaspoon of white wine vinegar and crack one or two eggs in to the pan. Immediately remove from the heat and cover. When the steak is cooked, let it rest on a warm plate until the eggs are poached (about three minutes). Eat at the table and imagine you are about to walk on the moon.

Mushroom omelette

Ingredients:
- Three fresh organic eggs.
- Some sliced organic mushrooms.
- Some organic butter.
- Sea salt and pepper.

Break three organic eggs into a bowl and beat gently with a fork. Season with salt and pepper. Melt a little organic butter in a small frying pan and gently sauté some sliced, organic mushrooms until they are soft. Pour in the eggs and when they start to set, tip the pan forward and 'push' the eggs into the middle of the pan with a spatula. Tip the pan backwards a little and 'pull' the egg mixture to the middle of pan again (if this technique is new to you, have a look in a good cookbook under 'How to cook the perfect omelette'). When the eggs are *just* still runny, fold over the omelette and tip onto a warm plate. Have a portion of 'Dave's One-Minute Wonder Salad' on the side for a delicious, healthy brunch or supper.

Kippers

I love kippers, but they can be a tricky to cook. Try this method:

Ingredients:
- One or two large kippers.
- One knob of butter.
- A slice of lemon.
- A tall Pyrex-type kitchen jug.
- Boiling water from the kettle.

Put the kippers 'head down' in the jug and cover with boiling water. Leave for about eight minutes, then remove and drain. Serve on a hot plate with a squeeze of lemon.

Scrambled eggs (with bacon or smoked salmon)

Very popular in our house, I make these all of the time. I

think I got the idea from Elizabeth David many years ago, but I suspect this is another generic recipe:

Ingredients:
- Two or three very fresh organic eggs.
- A knob of organic butter.
- Salt and white pepper.
- A good quality saucepan.
- A clear kitchen mixing bowl.
- Wooden spoon.

Crack the eggs into the mixing bowl, season with salt and white pepper and beat quickly with a fork. Melt butter in saucepan on a low heat. When butter is starting to foam, tip in the eggs and stir *continuously* with the wooden spoon. Now comes the tricky bit – eggs cook quickly and continue to cook when the pan is removed from the heat, so you have to anticipate a bit here. When the eggs just start to scramble, but *before* you think they are ready, remove the pan from the heat and keep stirring. Add another small knob of butter and another twist of white pepper. Then, another quick stir and you are done. Eat the eggs on their own (immediately or they will keep cooking and be ruined) or with some bacon perhaps (you can cook bacon in about two minutes in a microwave) or some beautiful sliced organic smoked salmon for a special treat.

Smoked haddock

Proper Grandma food, this! I was a bit suspicious about trying this recipe when I first discovered eating haddock in this way, but it is absolutely delicious. Don't be shy – try it for yourself and I promise you won't look back.

Ingredients:
- A nice fillet of smoked haddock (the *natural* smoked fish – not the artificial bright yellow variety).
- Some skimmed milk (as a special treat).
- A knob of organic butter.
- Salt and pepper.

Place the fish in a saucepan and cover with the milk. Add the butter and a twist of salt and pepper. Cover and cook *gently* for about ten minutes (if the heat is too high, the milk will boil over). Serve with loads of steam vegetables and have with a couple of poached eggs as a delicious brunch dish.

Dave's Kedgeree

I don't really allow rice on the Back to Basics programme because it is a processed carb. However, this dish makes a delicious weekend brunch and a bit of brown rice won't do you any harm, especially after your Sunday morning five-mile walk! This is my quick version of a classic recipe:

Ingredients:
- A small piece of smoked haddock.
- Two organic, free-range eggs.
- One medium onion, finely chopped.
- About half a litre of hot organic vegetable stock (made from stock powder).
- One teaspoon of mild curry powder and ½ teaspoon of turmeric.
- Half a pint of skimmed milk.
- Fresh parsley.
- Organic butter.
- Most of a small packet of organic brown basmati rice (about 300-400 grams).
- Fresh lemon and salt and pepper.

Cook the smoked haddock as per my earlier recipe. Boil the eggs in a saucepan of water until just hard-boiled (about eight minutes). Cook the onion in some butter until softened. Stir in the turmeric and curry powder and cook for one minute. Add the rice and stir thoroughly to coat each grain with the mixture. Add the stock and stir gently. Bring to the boil and turn the heat right down, cover and leave for about ten minutes. Check occasionally – cook until the rice is tender and all the liquid has been absorbed. Add more stock if necessary.

When the rice is cooked, remove skin (and any bones) from the smoked haddock and flake into bite-sized pieces with a fork. Peel the eggs and chop into small pieces as well.

Stir fish and eggs into the rice mixture and gently fold in. Warm through on the hob for a couple of minutes. Add some chopped parsley, a twist of salt and pepper and you're done. Serve with a large side salad. Delicious!

Quick and Easy dinners

Dave's Roast Chicken

This can be the centerpiece of any family meal. Remember to keep the carcass for making stocks and soups later on.

Ingredients:
* One or two fresh organic chickens.
* Some organic butter.
* An onion, peeled and cut in half.
* A selection of vegetables (e.g. carrots, cabbage, broccoli and cauliflower).
* Salt and pepper.

Take the chicken out of the fridge in good time (it needs to be at room temperature) and wash it inside and out under the tap. Put a bit of organic butter inside the cavity with the two onion halves and sprinkle a bit of sea salt and pepper over the skin. Roast at about 190C for twenty minutes to the pound plus twenty minutes. Make sure you baste regularly and you will end up with a perfect roast chicken. Steam the vegetables (I just put about half an inch of water in the bottom of a sauce pan, but you can buy a proper steamer if you wish) to preserve all the vitamins and phytonutrients – and there you have it. Add a portion of 'Dave's One-Minute Wonder Salad' and you have a delicious, healthy Sunday lunch for up to four people for less than the cost of eating out at a fast food restaurant.

Healthy chicken and vegetable soup

Ingredients:
- Some earthy vegetables (e.g. carrot, onion, celery, leek etc)
- Some fresh herbs (to your taste).
- Organic butter.
- An onion, peeled and cut in half.
- A bay leaf.
- Salt and pepper.
- A handful of red lentils.

Start by making a stock – fill a big saucepan with cold water and place the chicken carcass in the pan. Add a few earthy vegetables (e.g. a carrot, an onion cut in two, a piece of celery, maybe a leek). Add a little salt and pepper. Depending on your palate, you could try a few herbs in the stock as well. Bring to the boil, skim any 'scum' with a slotted spoon and then simmer for about two hours (put the lid on). Let the stock cool and then strain into a bowl or jug through a sieve (sounds complicated but it really isn't and if you do this when you first get home, it will be ready in time for dinner). Chop up some more vegetables (whatever you like, celery, onions, carrots etc) and 'sweat' them in a little butter in a saucepan for about twenty minutes. Add a little sea salt and pepper, pour in the stock, add a handful of red lentils and simmer for about twenty minutes. You can eat it as is or liquidise, as you wish.

Vegetable Curry

There is any number of recipes for a good curry, but this is my 'super-quick' version. You can make it in ten minutes, with a bit of practice.

Ingredients:
- Two or three onions.
- A tin of organic chickpeas.
- Assorted vegetables (e.g. celery, carrot, peas, runner beans, cauliflower).
- Cumin seeds.
- Cardamom pods.
- A clove of garlic, finely chopped.
- A piece of fresh ginger, finely chopped.
- A teaspoon of commercial curry powder.
- Rapeseed oil.
- Organic vegetable stock powder.
- Organic brown basmati rice, cooked as per instructions on the packet

First of all, roughly chop two or three onions, pop them in a saucepan, cover with boiling water from the kettle and bring to the boil. Turn the heat down and simmer for about seven minutes. Meanwhile, open a tin of organic chickpeas, chop up the veggies and put the whole lot in another saucepan, cover with boiling water and simmer until *just* soft (about five minutes). Drain when cooked. While the onions/vegetables are cooking, grind up the cumin seeds, cardamom pod, garlic, fresh ginger and curry powder (which can be mild, medium, hot, Madras etc, entirely up to you) in a pestle and mortar. When the onions are cooked, drain them and puree in a bowl with a handheld blender. Put a little rapeseed oil in the original pan and return to the heat – add the pureed onions and tip in the ground spice mixture from the pestle and mortar (eight minutes gone). Give the pan a stir and then mix up about a third of a pint of organic vegetable stock powder with boiling water from the kettle. Stir the drained veggies into the onion/spice pan. Add the vegetable stock. Cook for a further two minutes, check for seasoning and you are done. Have with a portion of organic brown basmati rice (the type you cook in a packet in a microwave will do, if necessary) and a large helping of my salad. Easy.

Dave's One-Minute Wonder Salad

Make this the basis of your meals by either having a large stand-alone portion for lunch or supper or a smaller portion as a side dish with your dinner. Take it to work in a plastic food box as well – just add a tin of tuna, some hard-boiled eggs or a piece of cold chicken for the perfect lunch, supper or office meal. You'll need to get a salad spinner to make salads from now on, but as you will be making them a lot, it is a sensible investment (try Lakeland – www.lakeland.co.uk). You can make this salad in one minute, provided everything is to hand in the kitchen.

Ingredients:
* Three teaspoons of organic extra virgin olive oil (from Crete).
* One teaspoon of white wine vinegar or lemon juice.
* ½ teaspoon of Dijon mustard (the smooth yellow variety, not the grainy one).
* Half a teaspoon of Himalayan salt and twist of black pepper.
* One cos (or Romaine) lettuce
* Tomatoes.
* Cucumber.
* A red onion.
* A packet of baby spinach.
* Some rocket.
* Fresh coriander.
* Any pre-cooked vegetables (e.g. cauliflower florets, broccoli etc).
* A tin of organic chickpeas

Start the clock ('tick, tock'). In a salad bowl, mix three teaspoons of Cretan extra virgin olive oil with *one* teaspoon of lemon juice or white wine vinegar. Stir in half a teaspoon of Dijon mustard. Add a twist of black pepper. Chop up a cos lettuce and chuck into your salad spinner. Rinse under the tap and spin vigorously! Thirty seconds gone! Tip the chopped-up lettuce into the salad bowl. Grab a kitchen knife and a chopping board (watch your fingers). Chop the following quickly and add to the salad bowl – some fresh tomatoes, half a cucumber, a red onion, some baby spinach (a packet?), some rocket (a packet?), some fresh coriander, any spare vegetables (e.g. some pre-cooked broccoli florets, cauliflower etc). Open a tin of organic chickpeas and tip some into the bowl (keep the rest for the curry). Mix thoroughly with your salad server spoons and that's it. Stop the clock – one minute up!

Gilly's Wonderful Asian Fish

My sister Gilly has long been cajoling me to eat more fish. She is the perfect example of why we should all eat fish on a regular basis – slim, fit, in perfect health and looking about twenty years younger than her true age. I'm not sure where she got this recipe (it is probably fairly generic), but it is easy and quick to make and absolutely delicious to boot. Try and source really fresh fish for this recipe – see my list of recommended suppliers in the Appendix. Serve with lots of steamed vegetables.

Ingredients:

- Fresh fillet of white fish (e.g. pla'
- Two spring onions, finely chopped.
- One clove of garlic, finely chopped.
- Some fresh ginger, finely chopped.
- One red chilli, finely chopped.
- Dash of rice wine.
- Dash of soy sauce.
- Dash of sesame oil.
- Twist of black pepper.
- A sheet of cooking foil.

Wash the fish and place in the centre of the foil. Cover with all the other ingredients. Fold the foil over the fish and scrunch up to make a sealed parcel. Place in fridge and leave to marinate overnight. When ready to cook, pre-heat oven to about 170C. Place foil parcel on baking tray and cook for twenty minutes. Be careful when opening the parcel not to scald yourself. Serve with steamed vegetables.

Quinoa and salad

I absolutely love quinoa and eat it about three times a week. It is one of the most nutritious of all vegetarian foods and is really versatile in terms of cooking and incorporating into other dishes. A very simple way to eat quinoa is to cook a portion and have it as a side dish, in lieu of potatoes or rice for instance.

redients:

A cup of organic quinoa (most supermarkets sell this nowadays).
- A teaspoon of organic vegetable stock powder.
- One medium onion, finely chopped.
- Some organic butter.
- About half a pint of boiling water from the kettle.
- One saucepan.

Melt some butter in the saucepan over a low heat and sauté the onion until soft. Tip the quinoa into the saucepan. Add about half a pint of boiling water from the kettle. Stir in a teaspoon of organic vegetable stock powder. Cover and cook gently until all the water is absorbed (about five minutes). Remove the lid and dry out the quinoa for a minute or so on a low heat. Fluff up with a fork and serve in a bowl. Try with Asian broccoli or a large 'Wonder' salad.

Tarka dall

I found this recipe on the Internet years ago, but I can't remember whose it was originally. If you're reading, please accept my apologies, but as it is such a good recipe, I would like your permission to repeat it here:

Ingredients:
- 9oz red lentils.
- 1.5 teaspoons ground cumin.

- Half a teaspoon turmeric.
- 1 teaspoon grated ginger (try 'very lazy ginger' in a jar from the supermarket).
- 1 red onion.
- Lots of chopped fresh coriander.
- 3 cloves garlic, finely chopped.
- Cumin seeds.
- Rapeseed oil.
- A suitable pan (a French cast iron elliptical pan is best).

Wash the lentils, then place in a pan on the hob with the ground cumin, grated ginger and 35fl oz boiling water. Bring to the boil and cook, uncovered, for twenty minutes. You will get a lot of yellow scum on the top – just scoop it off with a spoon. Then, turn heat down to lowest setting, put the lid on and leave for three hours.

After three hours, slice the red onion into very thin rounds and fry in a frying pan in the sunflower oil until caramalised. This is the crucial step – the onions should be almost burnt and give off a sort-of toffee flavour. Use a slotted spoon to collect onions (to drain the oil) and put into the lentil mixture. I add quite a large shot of salt, followed by the chopped coriander.

To finish, heat more oil in the same frying pan you used for the onions and sauté the garlic. As is starts to brown, bung in a goodly amount of cumin seeds. Fry for a minute and pour the whole mixture into the dall. Give it a very quick stir and then put the lid back on immediately to seal in the flavour. Serve hot with steamed vegetables and/or a *small* portion of organic brown basmati rice.

Salade Niçoise

A great classic French dish, suitable for either brunch or dinner. Enjoy with a glass of chilled rosé on a summer's day with friends and family and imagine you have been whisked away to the South of France.

Ingredients:
- One tin of tuna (in olive oil).
- A small tin of anchovies.
- Two fresh organic eggs.
- Two or three small new potatoes (for a special treat).
- Two tomatoes.
- A lettuce, washed.
- A handful of green beans ('haricots verts').
- A red onion, sliced into rings.
- Some black olives.
- Fresh basil.

In no particular order, boil the potatoes in a pan of water until cooked through. Cook the eggs until hard-boiled in a separate pan of water. Top and tail the beans and blanch them in a pan of salted, boiling water for only a minute. Drain and set aside. Mix up one serving of my vinaigrette in the bottom of a steep-sided salad bowl. Chop the lettuce and tomatoes and mix in the salad bowl with the olives and sliced red onion until fully coated with vinaigrette. Arrange the salad mixture on a large plate. Add the drained potatoes to the plate. Quickly sauté the blanched beans in a saucepan with a tablespoon of water and a knob of butter (for no more than a minute), then drain and add to the salad. Shell the eggs, cut into halves and place on the salad. Drain the tuna and place in the middle of the salad. Drain the anchovies and drape around the salad sporadically. Finally, sprinkle with chopped basil and pour over a little more vinaigrette over the whole salad – and voilà

My vinaigrette

This vinaigrette is a vital addition to many salads, including my Salade Niçoise.

Ingredients:
- Three spoonfuls of organic Cretan extra virgin olive oil.
- One spoonful of white wine vinegar.
- Teaspoon of Dijon mustard (the smooth yellow variety – not the grainy one).
- Half teaspoon of sea salt and twist of black pepper.

Mix all the ingredients together in the bottom of a deep wooden salad bowl. I use the back of a spoon to mix the mustard through thoroughly. Mix in a bowl and keep in a sealed jar in the fridge, though I just make it fresh each time I need it.

Asian broccoli

Use tenderstem broccoli and steam until just tender over a pan of boiling water. In another pan, gently sauté some sliced garlic in olive oil – but don't get the oil too hot or it will become unpleasant. When the broccoli is just cooked, tip it into the pan with the garlic and toss on a high heat for a minute or so. Add a dash of good quality soy sauce and serve immediately.

Dave's Famous Roast Pork

This is definitely a dish for a special occasion. I think it is better to avoid meat most of the time and eat vegetarian sources of protein, or chicken and fish. However, my wife loves this dish, so I make it now and again to keep her happy!

The secret to the perfect roast is to start with the best possible ingredients. That means making friends with your butcher or farm shop and getting hold of the best quality cut of meat you can. For this dish, my preference is for loin of pork on the bone, although belly of pork is also very tasty. Remember, this is the sort of 'centerpiece' meal that would be ideal for a family Sunday lunch or special occasion, where the leftovers can be used to make at least one, if not two, days' worth of tasty meals to follow. It is therefore quite expensive upfront but is actually a very economical way of eating, in line with dear old Grandma's theory.

Ingredients:

- One joint of free range loin of pork on the bone (try and source a rare breed such as Gloucester Old Spot).
- Some sea salt.
- A handful of sage.
- A large array of vegetables of your choice (e.g. cauliflower, carrots, broccoli, Savoy cabbage etc).
- A suitable pork stock cube.
- A hairdryer!

Take the joint out of the fridge in good time and turn the oven up to max. While the oven is heating up, plug your chosen hairdryer into a suitable socket in the kitchen. (Note for male chefs: If you are going to borrow said hairdryer from your wife, partner or mistress, I find it best to ask permission first! Oh, and make sure you wipe off any muck before handing it back – tends to make for a more pleasant ambience at dinner!)

Place joint in a suitable ovenproof roasting tin (the heavy cast iron French ones are best) and turn the hairdryer up to full. Play the hot air over the crackling for a few minutes, until the crackling is absolutely bone dry (ask your butcher to score the skin and 'chine' the joint when you buy). Once the oven is up to temperature and the crackling is dry, rub some crushed sea salt over the skin of the joint, sprinkle in a few sage leaves and place in the oven. Give it twenty minutes on max, then turn the heat down to about 190C (170C in a fan oven) and cook for thirty minutes per pound.

About twenty minutes from cooked, steam your choice of vegetables (lots) in a suitable steamer. When the pork is ready, take out of oven with oven gloves and transfer to a carving dish (use a two-pronged fork). Drain off most of the fat from the roasting tin and then place the roasting tin over a medium heat on the hob. Stir in some stock and some of the vegetable water (a slug of red wine is good, too) and reduce to a jus. Let the pork rest for a few minutes, then carve it up and serve with large chunks of perfect crackling. Enjoy with loads of vegetables and some jus. I don't like it, but most people would have some apple sauce with this as well.

Appendix 1

Basal Metabolic Rate (BMR)

One way we can clear up a common misunderstanding about our calorie requirements is to look at something called the Basal Metabolic Rate or BMR. Your BMR is a measure of the number of calories you need to keep you alive in any 24-hour day, before you do any exercise – in other words, the energy your body needs to keep functioning healthily. If you stayed in bed all day (alone!), you would pretty much burn up the calories as determined by your own BMR plus a bit, which varies in line with your age, sex, weight and height. Unfortunately, calculating your own BMR involves a rather scary sum. You don't have to do this, but it makes sense to establish your own BMR before going any further. How do we calculate our BMR? Grab a calculator and take a deep breath:

BASAL METABOLIC RATE

(Equations courtesy of www.bmi-calculator.net):

- For a woman, do this sum:
- 655 + (4.35 x your weight in pounds) + (4.7 x your height in inches) -- (4.7 x your age in years) = BMR
- For a man:
- 66 + (6.23 x your weight in pounds) + (12.7 x your height in inches) -- (6.8 x your age in years) = BMR
- As an example, imagine a 40-year-old female who is 65 inches tall and weighs 200lbs (14.3 stones). Crunching the numbers, the equation gives us a BMR of 1642. To relate this to 'normal' life, we have to do one more sum (something called the 'Harris Benedict' formula – please don't worry about it!). If our 40-year-old female is sedentary (i.e. does not take any regular exercise at all), we multiply the BMR by a factor of 1.2. So, 1642 x 1.2 = 1970 calories required for 'normal' life (let's call it 2000 calories to make the sums easier).
- This is now her true calorie requirement, which would allow her to maintain her current weight. To lose weight, she would need to eat slightly fewer calories or, better still, burn more calories each day though activity.

You can work out your own BMR, if you wish, to help you calculate an appropriate daily calorie intake. However, if you follow the advice and tips of the Back to Basics plan closely, you will *automatically* reduce your calorie consumption anyway. If you then take plenty of daily activity, you will easily expend more calories than you burn through exercise. With a bit of practice, you will soon find your own balance (how much to eat versus daily activity) to guarantee permanent weight loss.

Appendix 2

More details about the foods we eat

Meat

- Much of the meat offered to us today by the food industry is pretty dodgy, to be honest. Much mass-produced beef, for instance, involves cattle being cooped up in dark, cramped barns for large parts of the year before being fattened up on the fields for a couple of months each summer, prior to being dispatched to market.

- Although most of the beef production in this country is pretty good in terms of allowing the animals this sort of 'free range', they are still fed food supplements and doused with antibiotics to keep them well enough to get to market in sufficient quality to turn a profit. This is all a far cry from the sorts of meats our ancestors ate during our many thousands of years as hunter-gatherers.

- We have some wonderful organic farmers in the UK producing ethically-reared, high-quality meat at a fair price (see Appendix 3); however, there is an equally disturbing amount of evidence in the literature as to the potential health risks associated with eating red meat.

- Sadly, it seems there *is* a correlation between red meat consumption and certain cancers. The data is a bit 'hazy', as many of the people who appear to get ill from eating red meat also have significant other lifestyle issues, such as smoking, alcohol abuse, heavy consumption of burger buns and fries, together with the meat in the burgers.

- Nevertheless, the balance of evidence suggests we should give 'normal' red meat a wide berth most of the time, I'm afraid. If you stick to *natural* meat (e.g. hunt your own wild game or only ever eat *organic* or *biodynamic-produced* meat, for instance), you will probably never have a problem. In fact, you will almost certainly be a lot healthier than the vast majority of the population. All in all, though, try and eat vegetable proteins, organic poultry or fish in preference to most types of red meat as much as possible.

Fish

- The eating of fish has received a bad press in recent years. On one hand, we are told that fish are now so toxic because of heavy metal content (e.g. mercury) that we should avoid them at all costs. On the other hand, there are real concerns (which I wholly support) about the sustainability of various fish stocks around the World. Beyond these two issues, fish are an excellent source of healthy protein and fats. So, how on earth do we make sense of all this? Let me try and clear up some of these points as best I can.

- Firstly, I recommend eating certain types of fish on a regular basis. I personally enjoy eating fish and believe that if we are careful in our choices, fish provide us with a healthy and highly nutritious foodstuff. An excellent source of protein, many fish also provide high levels of very beneficial Omega 3 fatty acids.

- Nevertheless, there is no doubt that, until recently, we have made a complete mess of our stewardship of the World's oceans, rivers and larger areas of fresh water. For far too long and without appropriate controls, we have treated the seas and oceans as an indiscriminate dumping ground for our waste. Because the oceans are essentially 'out of sight and out of mind', the governments of the World have in the past turned a blind eye to their care and management, leading to large-scale pollution and the dumping of garbage.

- More recently though, it appears there are grounds for optimism. Various initiatives by organisations such as the Marine Stewardship Council (www.msc.org) and effective lobbying by various NGOs has led to a marked improvement in policy towards managing the oceans and associated fish stocks in a much more measured and proactive manner.

- There is still a lot more to do and we can all play our part by supporting groups that advocate good stewardship of our seas and rivers. In the UK, I recommend you consider joining and supporting the work of the Marine Conservation Society (www.mcsuk.org) or, worldwide, NGOs such as Greenpeace, Blue Ocean Institute, Oceana, The Ocean Conservancy and others, whose work is carefully focused on improving the lot of our wonderful seas and oceans.

- However, this doesn't help us much in terms of whether or not we should eat fish. Some fish definitely exhibit unsafe levels of heavy metal poisoning; as the Monterey Bay Aquarium in California, one of the World's finest marine organisations, says on their 'Seafood Watch' website: "Seafood contaminants include metals (such as mercury, which affects brain function and development), industrial chemicals (PCBs and dioxins) and pesticides (DDT). These toxins usually originate on land and make their way into the smallest plants and animals at the base of the ocean food web. As smaller species are eaten by larger ones, contaminants are concentrated and accumulated. Large predatory fish – like swordfish and shark – end up with the most toxins. You can minimise risks by choosing seafood carefully. Use our Super Green list and learn more about contaminants in seafood on the EDF website."

- So, we have to be careful in our fish choices due to concerns over toxins. However, we also have to consider that the World's oceans have been dramatically overfished for decades. Stocks of some species (e.g. North Sea cod) have almost completely collapsed due to overfishing.

- Nevertheless, as consumers, we can take a stand and demand that the fish we buy in the supermarkets and at the fishmongers comes from sustainable sources, which minimise the impacts on fish stocks and ease the pressure on already overstretched fisheries around the World.

Because there are so many local issues to do with fisheries management, I shall finish up this section with advice for UK shoppers trying to find healthy, sustainable sources of fresh fish. I will mention tinned fish in a moment. So, how should we in the UK source our fish? I suggest we try and do the following:

- Many of our supermarkets are making a real effort only to sell fish that comply with the MSC 'sustainable fishery' ethos. Marks and Spencer have probably taken this idea further than most, but they will never be the cheapest source of fish. Nevertheless, please support these initiatives and keep the pressure on, so that efforts continue to improve the sustainability of a wide range of fisheries.

- Have a look at the Greenpeace UK website (www.greenpeace.org.uk/oceans) for an excellent discussion of how to shop for sustainable fresh fish. In particular, please pay attention to their list of species to be avoided – unfortunately, this is now quite a long list, but I would certainly not purchase anything from the list. Neither should you.

- Although they would rather we didn't eat fish at all, Greenpeace recommend the best fish to purchase in the UK are line-caught mackerel and sea bass, purse-seined herring from Cornwall and farmed mussels. In this online age, I am perfectly happy to support good business that works to supply high-quality and sustainable fresh fish from around our coasts. I have no affiliation to these companies but I support both www.fishforthought.co.uk and Wing of St Mawes (www.thecornishfishmonger.co.uk) as reliable suppliers of high-quality fish. Check out Rick Steins website (www.rickstein.com/fish) for an expanded list of top-quality UK suppliers.

- Don't worry too much about toxins in fish. Just stay away from the large species where these toxins might accumulate (shark, swordfish etc) and eat fish just once or twice a week. I'm sure you will be fine. In fact, one of my favourite author's (Dr Steve Parker MD) claims to have never seen a single case of heavy metal poisoning from eating fish in his whole career.

- Stick to salmon, mackerel and sardines if eating tinned fish. Make sure you look for the MSC logo to ensure, as much as we can, that the fish is from sustainable sources. Please be careful when purchasing tuna; these magnificent animals are being hunted to extinction by mass fishing, so please ensure any tuna you buy is from sustainable (and dolphin-friendly) sources.

- In summary, I think that we should eat fish in moderation, thus providing us with an excellent source of protein and good fats. However, in this modern world, it is beholding on us all to ensure that we manage the oceans and their fish stocks properly for the benefit of future generations to come. Please try and play your part by shopping for fish in a sensible and ethical manner.

Dairy products:

- No other animal on this planet consumes milk other than from its mother during infancy. Humans are *unique* in drinking milk from other species of mammal.

- Prior to the invention of agriculture 10,000 years ago (and the domestication of cattle and goats), there would have been no source of dairy available to our hunter-gatherer ancestors. Can you imagine trying to milk a wild animal?

- Many of us today are *lactose-intolerant*. This is all to do with our genes, which still don't recognise the fact that we are consuming milk from another species.

- Yes, milk is full of protein and calcium, which is normally regarded as essential for good health and the avoidance of osteoporosis.

- However, recent research (see *The Greek Doctor Diet* by Dr Lindberg in the bibliography) refutes this idea. For instance, the Scandinavians consume high levels of milk but have the highest rates of osteoporosis in the world. By contrast, over a billion Chinese consume no dairy but suffer from extremely low rates of osteoporosis.

- The perceived benefit of calcium intake from milk seems to be largely exaggerated. Instead, a number of vitamins are involved in calcium uptake and retention, including Vitamin D and Vitamin K, which are best obtained from exposure to sunshine (Vitamin D) and from the consumption of leafy, green vegetables (Vitamin K).

- Add in some regular daily exercise and you have the solution to osteoporosis, without consuming unnatural dairy products.

Eggs

- Where do you think the consumption of eggs featured in the day-to-day diet of our *Paleo* ancestors? Pretty high up the list, I reckon.

- I haven't spent much time mired in 'egg literature' (honestly, I've got better things to do!), but I am fairly confident that the eggs of ground-laying birds would have provided an important source of food to our early ancestors.

- What about cholesterol? Well, there is little, if any, evidence of any disease in our pre-agricultural ancestors (or modern-day Aboriginal communities) caused by eating eggs. Instead, much current research is firmly in the 'eggs are a cheap, natural, nutritious food that are a good source of protein and vitamins' camp, rather than the largely outdated belief that eggs contain 'bad' cholesterol.

- Most researchers now accept that the cholesterol in eggs has virtually *no* impact at all on blood cholesterol levels. So, without going mad, feel free to include eggs in your new diet.

- I think a few eggs a week are fine; just make sure you choose *organic* eggs or, better still, get some chickens and have a fresh source of organic egg every morning. Please remember, though, that the risk of salmonella from eggs is still very real, so make sure you cook them properly.

Legumes

- Every schoolboy will titter at the mention of the dire effects we all experience from the overconsumption of pulses.

- However, those ghastly gaseous effects make sense in terms of our old friend the 'evolutionary perspective'.

- Has evolution designed us specifically to eat legumes? Don't think so. Has evolution equipped legumes with a suite of survival chemicals? Too right!

- In fact, most legumes contain a sugar called *oligosaccharide* that we can't digest. This leads to a bacterial explosion in our guts as our intestinal bacterial inhabitants feed off this unexpected sugar meal, producing their own 'mini-farts' by the trillion while they tuck into their free sugary lunch. We get to pay the price down the line.

- More importantly, though, legumes contain various chemical 'nasties', such as *lectin* (which we know causes leaky gut) and *phytoestrogens*, which interfere with the function of certain hormones.

- This all makes perfect sense to the accomplished legume chef because to make legumes palatable, we have to go through numerous stages of soaking, washing, rinsing, twice cooking, spicing and soaking again, just to be able to stomach them in our diet. I do eat *some* legumes and am particularly partial to Indian dall (lentils) and chickpeas prepared in numerous ways (including hummus, one of my favourite foods). However, I don't think legumes form a big part of our natural diet and I much prefer more *Paleo* foods, such as fruits and vegetables, fish, poultry, nuts, seeds and oils.

Appendix 3

Some recommended suppliers of 'real' foods

Meats and poultry:

- **Brown Cow Organics (www.browncoworganics.co.uk)** – one of the UK's best suppliers of organic beef. Highly recommended.
- **Heritage Prime (www.heritageprime.co.uk)** – supplies amazing biodynamic beef ('freezer'-sized orders only).
- **Higher Hacknell Farm (www.higherhacknell.co.uk)** – wonderful organic poultry, beef, pork and lamb. Home deliveries.
- **Laverstoke Park Farm (www.laverstokepark.co.uk)** – former racing driver Jody Scheckter's amazing biodynamic/organic farm in Hampshire. Wonderful range of products (chicken, beef etc), all home delivered.
- **Supermarkets** – most of the main supermarkets stock organic chickens. Do some research near your home and you will soon be able to source high-quality products.
- **Local butcher/Farmers' markets** – don't forget your local suppliers. If it proves hard to source organic poultry,

give them a hard time until they start stocking what you want. All power to the consumer!

Fish:

- **Martins Sea Fresh (www.martins-seafresh.co.uk)** – fantastic fish from Cornwall. Home deliveries.
- **Wing of St Mawes (www.cornishfishmonger.co.uk)** – another supplier of wonderful fresh seafood from Cornwall.
- **Whitby Seafish (www.whitbyseafish.co.uk)** – wonderful seafood and fish from Yorkshire.
- **Swallow Fish of Seahouses (www. swallowfish.co.uk)** – great smoked salmon and kippers from Northumberland.
- **L Robson and Sons (www.kipper.co.uk)** – the finest kippers from Craster, Northumberland.
- **Various supermarkets and fish vans** – most of the better supermarkets sell good quality fish these days. Keep your eye out for local fresh fish deliveries by the 'man in the van'. We get weekly visits from Fleetwood, which provide great fish at reasonable prices. Find out where you can buy such fish locally.

Fruit and veg

- Rather than list loads of suppliers here, I think it would be better if you located your own local organic fruit and vegetable producer. There are suitable growers all over the country now, but most only supply their local area. Join a box scheme or arrange a weekly delivery. Better still, try and grow your own.

Bibliography

Below is a list of various books, websites and blogs that I recommend you have a look at if you want to learn more about the fascinating world of human nutrition. I don't necessarily agree with all or any of these authors, so please approach with an open mind.

Gary Taubes (*Good Calories, Bad Calories*). Gary Taubes is a highly reputable science journalist who has thrown a major spanner into the 'diet-heart' hypothesis mainstream with this groundbreaking work. In a nutshell, Taubes provides (a huge amount) of evidence as to why he believes the 'low-fat, high-carbohydrate' dogma is wrong. Instead, he suggests an altered paradigm to a diet that is *low* in carbohydrate, not fat. His work has influenced many doctors, researchers, authors and bloggers (including me) and stands as a watershed in the rediscovery of the benefits of low-carb living.

Dr Joel Fuhrman (*Eat to Live*) – a highly eminent medical doctor who opened my eyes to the concept of nutrient density and the benefits of his 'Greens and Beans' diet.

Mark Sisson (www.marksdailyapple.com) – Mark Sisson is one of the leading lights in the 'Paleo' diet movement and his excellent blog is well worth reading on a regular basis.

Mark has really thrown the spotlight on the dangers of processed carbs in particular and has done a lot to improve the health of his many online followers.

Dr Steve Parker (www.diabeticmediterranean diet.com) – one of my favourite authors, Dr Parker has published a number of books about 'low-carb mediterranean diets' and runs an excellent blog, too. He is a highly experienced medical doctor who specialises in 'internal medicine' and the treatment of diabetics and obesity.

Dr John Mericle (www.micklediet.com) – Dr Mericle is an American doctor with strong views about vegan diets and intermittent fasting. An interesting read.

Professor Tim Noakes (http://thepaleodiet.co.za/professor-tim-noakes/) – Professor Noakes is a Professor of Sports Science at the University of Cape Town, South Africa and an acknowledged expert in the field of endurance sports and nutrition. A veteran of some seventy marathons and ultra-marathons himself, Professor Noakes wrote a famous book called *Lore of Running*, in which he espoused his then belief in the theories of 'carb loading' and high-carb diets. However, in recent years and in a quite remarkable turnaround (especially for such a well-known academic), he has completely changed his tune and now recommends a low-carbohydrate, high-protein diet instead.

Charles Dowding (www.charlesdowding.co.uk). Want to grow your own? I attended one of Charles's courses a few years ago and he remains an inspiration to those of us who want to successfully grow our own food at home or on the local allotment. A pioneer of the 'no dig' method of vegetable growing, Charles is a mine of information and an example to us all of why we should get out in the garden and plant something. He has certainly helped me get the 'bug' for growing my own veg – there's nothing like it.

References

Introduction

1. WHO (World Health Organization). (2000) *Obesity: preventing and managing the global epidemic*. WHO technical report series 894.
    Wang YC, McPherson K, Marsh T, Gortmaker SL,
2. Brown M. (2011) 'Health and economic burden of the projected obesity trends in the USA and the UK'. *The Lancet,* 378, pp. 815-825.
3. WHO (World Health Organization). (March 2013) 'Obesity and overweight', Fact sheet N°311.
4. The Health & Social Care Information Centre (HSCIC). (December 2012) 'Health Survey for England – 2011, Health, social care and lifestyles [NS]'.
5. The Health & Social Care Information Centre (HSCIC). (2012) 'Statistics on obesity, physical activity and diet: England, 2012'.
6. Wang, Y. and Beydoun, MA. (2007). 'The obesity epidemic in the United States—gender, age, socioeconomic, racial/ethnic, and geographic characteristics: a systematic review and meta-regression analysis', *Epidemiol Rev,* 29, 6-28.
7. Wang, Y., Beydoun, M.A., Liang, L., Cabellero, B. and Kumanyika, SK. (2008) 'Will All Americans Become Overweight or Obese? Estimating the Progression and Cost

of the US Obesity Epidemic', *Obesity,* 16 (10), 2323-2330.

8. Whitlock, G. et al. (2009) 'Body-mass index and cause-specific mortality in 900 000 adults: collaborative analyses of 57 prospective studies', *The Lancet,* 28; 373(9669).

9. Chauhan, H.K. (2012) 'Diabesity: the 'Achilles Heel' of our modernized society'. *Rev Assoc Med Bras,* 2012 Jul-Aug; 58(4): 399.

10. Morgan, E. and Dent, M. (2010). *'The economic burden of obesity'*, Oxford: The National Obesity Observatory.

11. The Health and Social Care Information Centre (HSCIC). (2013) 'Statistics on obesity, physical activity and diet: England, 2013.'

12. Ogden, C.L., Carroll, M.D., Curtin, L.R., McDowell, M.A., Tabak, C.J. and Flegal, K.M. (2006) 'Prevalence of overweight and obesity in the United States, 1999-2004', *Jama,* 295 (13): 1549–55.

13. US Department of Health and Human Services. (2000) 'Healthy people 2010', 2nd ed. Washington, DC: US Government Printing Office.

14. Aggarwal, A., Monsivais, P., Cook, A.J. and Drewnowski, A. (2011) 'Does diet cost mediate the relation between socioeconomic position and diet quality? *European Journal of Clinical Nutrition.*

15. Brooks, R.C., Simpson, S.J., Raubenheimer, D. (2010) 'The price of protein: combining evolutionary and economic analysis to understand excessive energy consumption'. *Obes Rev.* 11(12): 887-894.

16. Prentice, A.M. and Jebb, S.A. (2003) 'Fast foods, energy density and obesity: a possible mechanistic link', *Obes Rev.* 4:187-194.

17. Aggarwal, A., Monsivais, P., Cook, A.J. and Drewnowski, A.

(2011) 'Does diet cost mediate the relation between socioeconomic position and diet quality?' *European Journal of Clinical Nutrition.*

Part One
Chapter 1

1. Bloch Eidner, M. et al. (2013) 'Calories and portion sizes in recipes throughout 100 years: An overlooked factor in the development of overweight and obesity?' *Scand J Public Health.*
2. Sikorski, C. et al. (2012) 'Obese children, adults and senior citizens in the eyes of the general public: results of a representative study on stigma and causation of obesity', *PLoSOne,* 7(10) e46924.
3. Mozaffarian, D. et al. (2011) 'Changes in Diet and Lifestyle and Long-Term Weight Gain in Women and Men', *N Engl J Med*, 364(25): 2392–2404.
4. Bomstein, S.R. et al. (2008) 'Is the worldwide epidemic of obesity a communicable feature of globalization?' *Exp Clin Endocrinol Diabetes,* 116 Suppl 1:S30-2.
5. Zilberter, T. (2012) 'Food Addiction and Obesity: Do Macronutrients Matter?' *Front Neuroenergetics,* 4:7.
6. Prentice & Jebb. (1995) 'Gluttony or sloth?' *BMJ*, 311, 437.
7. Jew, S. et al. (2009) 'Evolution of the human diet: linking our ancestral diet to modern functional foods as a means of chronic disease prevention', *J Med Food*, 12(5):925-34.
8. Russell-Jones, D. and Khan, R. (2007) 'Insulin-associated weight gain in diabetes—causes, effects and coping strategies', *Diabetes Obes Metab,* 9(6):799-812.
9. Despres, J.P. (1993) 'Abdominal obesity as important

component of insulin-resistance syndrome', *Nutrition,* 1993;9:452–459.

10. Weiss, R. et al. (2013) 'What is metabolic syndrome, and why are children getting it?', *Ann. N.Y. Acad. Sci,* ISSN 0077-8923

11. Frassetto, L.A., Schloetter, M., Mietus-Synder, M., Morris, R.C. Jr, and Sebastian, A. (2009). Metabolic and physiologic improvements from consuming a paleolithic, hunter-gatherer type diet. *Eur J Clin Nutr,* 63(8):947–955.

12. Newby, P.K., Muller, D., Hallfrisch, J. et al. (2003) 'Dietary patterns and changes in body mass index and waist circumference in adults', *Am J Clin Nutr,* 77:1417–1425.

Chapter 2

1. Puhl, R.M. et al. (2013) 'Weight bias among professionals treating eating disorders: Attitudes about treatment and perceived patient outcomes', *Int J Eat Disord* 10.1002/eat.22186.

2. Vadiveloo, M. et al. (2013) 'Trends in dietary fat and high-fat food intakes from 1991 to 2008 in Framingham Heart Study participants', *Br J Nutr Sep* 19:1-11.

3. Volger, S. et al. (2013) 'Changes in eating, physical activity and related behaviors in a primary care-based weight loss intervention', *Int J Obes (Lond)* 37 Suppl 1:S12-8.

4. Sparling, P.B. et al. (2013) 'Energy balance: the key to a unified message on diet and physical activity', *J Cardiopulm Rehabil Prev,* 33(1): 12-5.

5. Buchholz, A.C. and Schoeller, D.A. (2004) 'Is a calorie a calorie?' *Am J Clin Nutr,* 79(5):899S-906S.

6. Feinman, R.D., Fine, E.J. (2004) 'Whatever happened to the

second law of thermodynamics?' *Am J Clin Nutr,* 80(5):1445-6.

7. Schwarzfuchs, D. and Golan, R. (2012) 'Four-Year Follow-up after Two-Year Dietary Interventions', *N Engl J Med,* 367:1373-1374.

8. Pereira, H.R. et al. (2013) 'Childhood and adolescent obesity: how many extra calories are responsible for excess of weight?' *Rev Paul Paediatr,* 31(2): 252-7.

9. Slyper, A.H. (2013) 'The influence of carbohydrate quality on cardiovascular disease, the metabolic syndrome, type 2 diabetes, and obesity – an overview', *J Paediatr Endocrinol Metab,* 26(7-8): 617-29.

10. Troesch, B. et al. (2012) 'Dietary surveys indicate vitamin intakes below recommendations are common in representative Western countries', *Br J Nutr,* 108(4):692-8.

11. Cizzer, G. and Rother, K.I. (2012) 'Beyond fast food and slow motion: weighty contributors to the obesity epidemic', *J Endocrinol Invest,* 35(2): 236-42.

12. Srinivasan, C.S. (2013) 'Can adherence to dietary guidelines address excess caloric intake? An empirical assessment for the UK', *Econ Hum Biol,* S1570-677X(13)00038-5.

13. Anton, S. and Leeuwenburgh, C. (2013) 'Fasting or caloric restriction for Healthy Aging', *Exp Gerontol,* 48(10): 1003-5.

Chapter 3

1. Schell, L.M. et al. (2012) 'What's NOT to eat – Food adulteration in the context of human biology', *Am J Hum Biol,* 24(2): 139-148.

2. Diamond, J. (1987) 'The Worst Mistake In The History Of The Human Race', *Discover,* pp. 64-66.

3.   Milton, K. (2002) 'Hunter-gatherer diets: wild foods signal relief from diseases of affluence' in *Human Diet: Its Origins and Evolution*, ed. by Peter Ungar and Mark Teaford, Westport, CT Bergin & Garvey, pp. 111-122.

4.   Gunz, P. et al. (2009) 'Early modern human diversity suggests subdivided population structure and a complex out-of-Africa scenario', *Proc Natl Acad Sci U S A* 106(15): 6094–6098.

5.   Cartmill, M. et al. (2009) *The human lineage*, New York: John Wiley.

6.   Strait, D.S. et al. (2009) 'The feeding biomechanics and dietary ecology of *Australopithecus africanus*', *Proc Natl Acad Sci U S A*, 106 (7).

7.   Tattersall, I. (2009) 'Human origins: Out of Africa', *Proc Natl Acad Sci U S A,* 106(38): 16018-16021.

8.   Wolpoff, M.H., Hawks, J., Frayer, D.W. and Hunley, K. (2001) 'Modern human ancestry at the peripheries: A test of the replacement theory', *Science*, 291:293-297.

9.   Stringer, C. and McKie, R. (1996) *African Exodus: The Origins of Modern Humanity*, New York: Henry Holt.

10. Antón, S.C. (2003) 'Natural history of Homo erectus', *Yearbook of Physical Anthropology*, 46:126-170.

11. Carrera-Bastos, P. et al. (2011) 'The western diet and lifestyle and diseases of civilization', *Research Reports in Clinical Cardiology* 2011:2.

12. Milton, K. (2000) 'Back to basics: why foods of wild primates have relevance for modern human health', *Nutrition,* 16:481-483.67.

13. Milton, K. (2000) 'Hunter-gatherer diets: a different perspective', *American Journal of Clinical Nutrition,* 71:665-6000.

14. Chatzi, L. et al. (2007) 'Protective effect of fruits, vegetables

and the Mediterranean diet on asthma and allergies among children in Crete', *Thorax,* 62(8): 677–683.

15. Cordain, L., Eaton, S.B., Sebastian, A., Mann, N., Lindeberg, S., Watkins, B.A., O'Keefe, J.H. and Brand-Miller, J. (2005) 'Origins and evolution of the western diet: Health implications for the 21st century', *Am J Clin Nutr,* 81:341-54.

16. Diamond, J. et al. (2003) 'Farmers and Their Languages: The First Expansions', *Science,* 300, 597; DOI: 10.1126/science.1078208.

17. Barrett, S.C.H. (2010) 'Darwin's legacy: The forms, function and sexual diversity of flowers', *Philos Trans R Soc Lond B Biol Sci.*; 365(1539): 351–368.

18. De Punder, K. and Pruimboom, L. (2013) 'The Dietary Intake of Wheat and other Cereal Grains and Their Role in Inflammation', *Nutrients* 2013, *5,* 771-787.

19. Eaton, S.B. (2006) 'The ancestral human diet: what was it and should it be a paradigm for contemporary nutrition?' *Proc Nutr Soc,* 65(1): 1-6.

20. McPherron, S.P., Alemseged, Z., Marean, C.W., Wynn, J.G., Reed, D., Geraads, D., Bobe, R. and Bearat, H.A. (2010) 'Evidence for stone-tool-assisted consumption of animal tissues before 3.39 million years ago at Dikika, Ethiopia', *Nature,* 466 (7308): 857-860.

Chapter 4

1. Prentice & Jebb (2007) 'Fast foods, energy density and obesity: a possible mechanistic link', *Obesity Reviews,* 4, 187.

2. Bremer, A.A. et al. (2012) 'Towards a Unifying Hypothesis of Metabolic Syndrome', *Pediatrics,* 129(3): 557–570.

3. Valenzuela, R.E.R. et al. (2013) 'Insufficient amounts and inadequate distribution of dietary protein intake in apparently healthy older adults in a developing country: implications for dietary strategies to prevent sarcopenia', *Clinical Interventions in Aging*, 2013:8.

4. Galperin, M.Y. and Koonin, U.V. (2012) 'Divergence and Convergence in Enzyme Evolution', *J Biol Chem*, 287(1): 21–28.

5. Segasothy, M. and Phillips, P.A. (1999) 'Vegetarian diet: panacea for modern lifestyle diseases?', *QJM*, 92(9):531-44.

6. Martin-Peláez et al (2013) 'Health effects of olive oil polyphenols: recent advances and possibilities for the use of health claims', *Mol Nutr Food Res*, 57(5):760-71.

7. Taubes, G. (2008) *Good Calories, Bad Calories: Fats, carbs and the controversial science of Diet and health*, Anchor.

8. Keys, A. (1970) 'Coronary heart disease in seven countries', *Circulation*, 41 supplement 1: 1-1 through 1-211.

9. Keys, A. (1980) *Seven countries: A multivariate analysis of death and coronary heart disease*, Harvard University press.

10. Cordain, L. (2006) 'Saturated fat consumption in ancestral human diets: implications for contemporary intakes' in *Phytochemicals, Nutrient-Gene Interactions*, ed. by Meskin, M.S., Bidlack, W.R., Randolph, R.K, CRC Press (Taylor & Francis Group), pp. 115-126.

11. Catlin, G. (1844) *Letter and notes on the Manners, Customs and Conditions of North American Indians Vol 1 and 2*, New York: Dover Pubs, reprinted 1971.

12. German, J.B. and Dillard, C.J. (2004) 'Saturated fats: what dietary intake?' *Am J Clin Nutr*, 80:550-559.

13. Forsythe, C.E. et al. (2010) 'Limited effect of dietary saturated

fat on plasma saturated fat in the context of a low carbohydrate diet', *Lipids,* 45(10):947-62.

14. Wainwright, P.E. (2002) 'Dietary essential fatty acids and brain function: a developmental perspective on mechanisms', *Proc Nutr Soc,* 61(1):61-9.

15. Apte, S.A. et al. (2013) 'A low dietary ratio of omega-6 to omega-3 Fatty acids may delay progression of prostate cancer', *Nutr Cancer,* 65(4):556-62.

16. Choque, B. et al. (2013) 'Linoleic acid: Between doubts and certainties', *Biochimie,* S0300-9084(13)00234-4.

17. Simopoulos, A.P. (2002) 'The importance of the ratio of omega-6/omega-3 essential fatty acids', *Biomed Pharmacother* 56(8):365-79.

18. Brouwer, I.A. et al. (2013) 'Trans fatty acids and cardiovascular health: research completed?' *Eur J Clin Nutr,* 67(5):541-7.

19. Jaworowska, A. et al. (2013) 'Nutritional challenges and health implications of takeaway and fast food', *Nutr Rev,* 71(5):310-8.

20. Dyson, P.A. et al. (2007) 'A low-carbohydrate diet is more effective in reducing body weight than healthy eating in both diabetic and non-diabetic subjects', *Diabet Med,* 24(12):1430-5.

21. Feinman, R.D. and Volek, J.S. (2008) 'Carbohydrate restriction as the default treatment for type 2 diabetes and metabolic syndrome', *Scand Cardiovasc J,* 42:256-26.

22. Westman, E.C. (2002) 'Is dietary carbohydrate essential for human nutrition?' *The American journal of clinical nutrition,* 75 (5): 951–3.

23. Aller, E.J.G. et al. (2011) 'Starches, Sugars and Obesity', *Nutrients,* 3(3): 341-369.

24. Fuhrman, J. (2003) *Eat to live. The revolutionary Formula for Fast and Sustained Weight Loss*, Little Brown & Company, 1st edition.

25. Malik, V.S., Popkin, B.M., Bray, G.A., Després, J.P. and Hu, F.B. (2010) 'Sugar-sweetened beverages, obesity, type 2 diabetes mellitus and cardiovascular disease risk', *Circulation*, 121(11):1356–1364.

26. Jenkins, D.J., Wolever, T.M., Taylor, R.H., Barker, H., Fielden, H. et al. (1981) 'Glycemic index of foods: a physiological basis for carbohydrate exchange', *Am J Clin Nutr*, 34: 362-366.

27. Barclay, A.W., Petocz, P., McMillan-Price, J et al. (2008) 'Glycemic index, glycemic load, and chronic disease risk—a meta-analysis of observational studies', *Am J Clin Nutr*, 87:627-637.

Chapter 5

1. Marlowe, F.W. (2005) 'Hunter-gatherers and human evolution', *Evol Anth*, 14:54-67.

2. Pontzer, H., Raichlen, D.A., Wood, B.M., Mabulla, A.Z.P., Racette, S.B. et al. (2012) 'Hunter-Gatherer Energetics and Human Obesity', *PLoS ONE* **7** (7): e40503.

3. Popkin, B.M. et al. (2013) 'NOW AND THEN: The Global Nutrition Transition: The Pandemic of Obesity in Developing Countries', *Nutr Rev*, 70 (1): 3-21.

4. Williams, D.L. and Schwarz, M.W. (2011) 'Neuroanatomy of body weight control: lessons learned from leptin', *J Clin Invest*, 121(6): 2152–2155.

5. Conte, C. et al. (2012) 'Multiorgan Insulin Sensitivity in Lean and Obese Subjects', *Diabetes Care*, 35(6): 1316-1321.

6. Musselman, L.P. et al. (2011) 'A high-sugar diet produces

obesity and insulin resistance in wild-type Drosophila, *Dis Model Mech,* 4(6): 842–849.

7. Shapiro, A., Mu, W., Roncal, C., Cheng, K.Y., Johnson, R.J. and Scarpace, P.J. (2008) 'Fructose-induced leptin resistance exacerbates weight gain in response to subsequent high-fat feeding', *Am J Physiol Regul Integr Comp Physiol*, 295, R1370-1375.

8. Taubes, G. (2010) *Why we get fat and what to do about it,* New York: Knopf.

9. Cizza, G. and Rother, K.I. (2012) 'Beyond fast food and slow motion: Weighty contributors to the obesity epidemic', *J Endocrinol Invest,* 35(2): 236-242.

10. Frederich, R.C., Hamann, A., Anderson, S., Lollmann, B., Lowell, B.B. and Flier, J.S. (1995) 'Leptin levels reflect body lipid content in mice: evidence for diet-induced resistance to leptin action', *Nat Med*, 1:1311-1314.

11. Zhang, Y., Proenca, R., Maffei, M., Barone, M., Leopold, L. and Friedman, J.M. (1994) 'Positional cloning of the mouse obese gene and its human homologue', *Nature,* 372:425-432.

12. Boden, G. (2011) 'Obesity, insulin resistance and free fatty acids', *Current opinion in endocrinology, diabetes, and obesity*, 18:139-143.

13. Kahn, S.E., Hull, R.L. and Utzschneider, K.M. (2006) 'Mechanisms linking obesity to insulin resistance and type 2 diabetes', *Nature,* 444:840-846.

14. Rui, L. (2013) 'Brain regulation of energy balance and body weight', *Rev Endocr Metab Disord*, Aug 30.

15. Centers for Disease Control and Prevention (CDC), 'Overweight and obesity'; 'Childhood overweight and obesity'.

16. Dyson, P.A. et al. (2007) 'A low-carbohydrate diet is more effective in reducing body weight than healthy eating in both diabetic and non-diabetic subjects', *Diabet Med,* 24(12): 1430-5.

17. Guyton, A.C and Hall, J.E. (2006) 'Chapter 78: Insulin, Glucagon, and Diabetes Mellitus' in *Textbook of Medical Physiology* (11th ed.), Philadelphia: Elsevier Saunders, pp. 963-68.

18. Kahn, B.B. and Flier, S.S. (2000) 'Obesity and insulin resistance', *J Clin Invest,* 106(4): 473-481.

19. Chakrabarti, P. et al. (2013) 'Insulin Inhibits Lipolysis in Adipocytes via the Evolutionarily Conserved mTORC1-Egr1-ATGL-Mediated Pathway', *Mol Cell Biol,* 33(18):3659-66.

20. Wilcox, G. (2005) 'Insulin and Insulin Resistance', *Clin Biochem Rev*, 26(2): 19-39.

21. El Khatib, H.F. et al. (2007) 'Adaptive Closed-Loop Control Provides Blood-Glucose Regulation Using Dual Subcutaneous Insulin and Glucagon Infusion in Diabetic Swine', *J Diabetes Sci Technol*, 1(2): 181-192.

22. Tsatsoulis, A. et al. (2013) 'Insulin resistance: an adaptive mechanism becomes maladaptive in the current environment – an evolutionary perspective', *Metabolism*, 62(5):622-33.

23. Hansen, M., Chandra, A., Mitic, L.L., Onken, B., Driscoll, M. and Kenyon, C. (2008) 'A role for autophagy in the extension of lifespan by dietary restriction' in *Caenorhabditis elegans*, *PLoS Genetics* 4(2):e24.

24. Hsu, A.L., Murphy, C.T. and Kenyon, C. (2003) 'Regulation of aging and age-related disease by DAF-16 and Heat-Shock Factor', *Science* 300 (5622), 1142-1145.

25. Kui Lin, Hsin, H., Libina, N. and Kenyon, C. (2001) 'Regulation of the *Caenorhabditis elegans* longevity protein

DAF-16 by insulin/IGF-1 and germline signaling', *Nature Genetics,* 28(2), 139-145.

Chapter 6

1. Ravnskov, U. (1998) 'The questionable role of saturated and polyunsaturated fatty acids in cardiovascular disease', *J Clin Epidemiol,* 51:443-460.
2. Pavitt, Nigel. (1997) *'Turkana'*, London: Harvill Press.
3. Lindeberg, S., Nilsson-Ehle, P., Terént, A., Vessby, B. and Scherstén, B. (1994) 'Cardiovascular risk factors in a Melanesian population apparently free from stroke and ischaemic heart disease – the Kitava study', *J Intern Med,* 236: 331-340.
4. Popkin, B.M., Adair, L.S. and Ng, S.W. (2012) 'Global nutrition transition and the pandemic of obesity in developing countries', *Nutr Rev,* **70**:3-21.
5. Zheng, W. et al. (2011) 'Association between body-mass index and risk of death in more than 1 million Asians', *N Engl J Med,* 364(8):719-729.
6. Mehio Sibai, A., Nasreddine, L., Mokdad, A.H., Adra, N., Tabet, M. and Hwalla, N. (2010) 'Nutrition transition and cardiovascular disease risk factors in Middle East and North Africa countries: reviewing the evidence', *Ann Nutr Metab,* 57(3-4).
7. Volek, J.S. (2012) 'Carbohydrate restriction uniquely benefits metabolic syndrome and saturated fat metabolism', *BMC Proc,* 6(Suppl 3).
8. Spreadbury, I. (2012) 'Comparison with ancestral diets suggests dense acellular carbohydrates promote an inflammatory microbiota, and may be the primary dietary cause of leptin

resistance and obesity', *Diabetes Metab Syndr Obes*, 5:175-89.

9. Lindeberg, S., Soderberg, S., Ahren, B. and Olsson, T. (2001) 'Large differences in serum leptin levels between nonwesternized and westernized populations: the Kitava study', *J Intern Med*, **249**(6):553-558.

10. Frassetto, L.A., Schloetter, M., Mietus-Synder, M., Morris, R.C. Jr and Sebas- tian, A. (2009) 'Metabolic and physiologic improvements from consuming a paleolithic, hunter-gatherer type diet', *Eur J Clin Nutr*, **63**(8): 947-955.

11. Lassenius, M.I., Pietilainen, K.H., Kaartinen, K. et al. (2011) 'Bacterial endotoxin activity in human serum is associated with dyslipidemia, insulin resistance, obesity, and chronic inflammation', *Diabetes Care*, **34**(8): 1809-1815.

12. Vessby, B., Ahren, B., Warensjo, E. and Lindgarde, F. (2012) 'Plasma lipid fatty acid composition, desaturase activities and insulin sensitivity in Amerindian women', *Nutr Metab Cardiovasc Dis*, 22(3):176-181.

13. Carvalho, B.M. and Saad, M.J. (2013). 'Influence of gut microbiota on subclinical inflammation and insulin resistance', *Mediators Inflamm*, 2013:986734.

14. Draznin, B. (2006) 'Molecular mechanisms of insulin resistance: serine phosphorylation of insulin receptor substrate-1 and increased expression of p85alpha: the two sides of a coin', *Diabetes,* 55(8):2392-7.

15. Marini, M.A. et al. (2013) 'Differences in insulin clearance between metabolically healthy and unhealthy obese subjects', *Acta Diabetol*, Aug 30.

16. Shanik, M.H. et al. (2008) 'Insulin resistance and hyperinsulinemia: is hyperinsulinemia the cart or the horse?' *Diabetes Care*, 31 Suppl 2:S262-8.

17. World Health Organization (WHO). (2006) *Definition and diagnosis of diabetes mellitus and intermediate hyperglycemia: report of a WHO/IDF consultation*, Geneva: World Health Organization, p. 21.

18. Farooqi, I.S., Bullmore, E., Keogh, J., Gillard, J., O'Rahilly, S., Fletcher, P.C. (2007) 'Leptin regulates striatal regions and human eating behavior', *Science*. 317:1355.

Chapter 7

1. http://www.livestrong.com/article/40956-six-small-meals-day-diet/

2. Cameron, J.D., Cyr, M.J. and Doucet, E. (2010) 'Increased meal frequency does not promote greater weight loss in subjects who were prescribed an 8-week equi-energetic energy-restricted diet', *Br J Nutr*, *103*(8):1098-101.

3. DeBerardinis, R.J. and Craig, B.T. (2012) 'Cellular metabolism and disease: what do metabolic outliers teach us?' *Cell*, 148(6): 1132-1144.

4. Solomon, T.P.J. et al. (2008) 'The effect of feeding frequency on insulin and ghrelin responses in human subjects', *British Journal of Nutrition*, 100, 810-819.

5. Oh, K.J. et al. (2013) 'Transcriptional regulators of hepatic gluconeogenesis', *Arch Pharm Res*. **36**(2):189-200.

6. Nishino, N. et al. (2007) 'Insulin Efficiently Stores Triglycerides in Adipocytes by Inhibiting Lipolysis and Repressing PGC-1 Induction', *Kobe J. Med. Sci*, Vol. 53, No. 3, pp. 99-106.

7. Bonadonna, R.C., Groop, L.C., Zych, K., Shank M. and DeFronzo, R.A. (1990) 'Dose-dependent effect of insulin

on plasma free fatty acid turnover and oxidation in humans', *Am. J. Physiol,* 259(Endocrinol. Metab. 22):E736-E750.

8. Campbell, P.J., Carlson, M.G., Hill, J.O. and Nurjhan, N. (1992) 'Regulation of free fatty acid metabolism by insulin in humans: role of lipolysis and reesterification', *Am. J. Physiol,* 263(Endocrinol. Metab. 26):E1063-E1069.

9. Berg, J.M., Tymoczko, J.T. and Stryer, L. (2002) *Biochemistry,* (5th edition), New York: W H Freeman.

10. Chambliss, H.O. (2005) 'Exercise duration and intensity in a weight-loss program', *Clin J Sport Med*, 15(2):113-5.

11. Nematy, M. et al (2012). Effects of Ramadan fasting on cardiovascular risk factors: a prospective observational study. *Nutr J.* **11**: 69.

12. Shariatpanahi, Z.V., Shariatpanahi, M.V., Shahbazi, S., Hossaini, A. and Abadi, A. (2008) 'Effect of Ramadan fasting on some indices of insulin resistance and components of the metabolic syndrome in healthy male adults', *Br J Nutr,* 100(1):147-151.

13. Bouguerra, R., Jabrane, J., Maatki, C., Ben, S.L., Hamzaoui, J., El, K.A. et al. (2006) 'Ramadan fasting in type 2 diabetes mellitus', *Ann Endocrinol* **67**(1):54-59.

Part Two
Chapter 10

1. Agudo, A., Slimani, N., Ocké, M.C. et al. (2002) 'Consumption of vegetables, fruit and other plant foods in the European prospective investigation into cancer and nutrition

(EPIC) cohorts from 10 European countries', *Public Health Nutr*, 5:1179-1196.

2. Alinia, S., Hels, O. and Tetens, I. (2009) 'The potential association between fruit intake and body weight – a review', *Obes Rev*, 10:639-647.

3. Appleby, P.N., Thorogood, M., Mann, J.I. and Key, T.J. (1999) 'The Oxford Vegetarian Study: an overview', *Am J Clin Nutr,* 70 (3 Suppl): 525S-531S.

4. Bazzano, L.A. (2005) 'Dietary intake of fruits and vegetables and risk of diabetes mellitus and cardiovascular disease', Geneva: World Health Organization.

5. Bendinelli, B., Masala, G., Saieva, C. et al. (2011) 'Fruit, vegetables, and olive oil and risk of coronary heart disease in Italian women: the EPICOR Study' *Am J Clin Nutr*. **93**:275–283.

6. Block, G., Patterson, B. and Subar, A. (1992) 'Fruit, vegetables, and cancer prevention: a review of the epidemiological evidence', *Nutr Cancer*, 18: 29.

7. Boffetta, P., Couto, E., Wichmann, J. et al. (2010) 'Fruit and vegetable intake and overall cancer risk in the European Prospective Investigation into Cancer and Nutrition (EPIC)', *J Natl Cancer Inst*, 102:529-537.

8. Buijsse, B., Feskens, E.J., Schulze, M.B. et al. (2009) 'Fruit and vegetable intakes and subsequent changes in body weight in European populations: results from the project on diet, obesity, and genes (DiOGenes)', *Am J Clin Nutr*, 90:202-209.

9. Carter, P., Gray, L.J., Troughton, J. et al (2010) 'Fruit and vegetable intake and incidence of type 2 diabetes mellitus: systematic review and meta-analysis', *BMJ*, 341:c4229.

10. Crowe, F.L., Roddam, A.W., Key, T.J. et al. (2011) 'European prospective investigation into cancer and nutrition (EPIC)-

heart study collaborators. Fruit and vegetable intake and mortality from ischaemic heart disease: results from the European Prospective Investigation into Cancer and Nutrition (EPIC)-Heart Study', *Eur Heart J*, 32:1235-1243.

11. Dauchet, L., Amouyel, P. and Dallongeville, J. (2005) 'Fruit and vegetable consumption and risk of stroke: a metaanalysis of cohort studies', *Neurology* 65: 1193-1197.

12. Dauchet, L., Amouyel, P., Hercberg, S. and Dallongeville, J. (2006) 'Fruit and vegetable consumption and risk of coronary heart disease: a meta-analysis of cohort studies', *J Nutr*, 136: 2588-2593.

13. Davey, G.K., Spencer, E.A., Appleby, P.N., Allen, N.E., Knox, K.H. and Key, T.J. (2003) 'EPIC-Oxford: lifestyle characteristics and nutrient intakes in a cohort of 33 883 meat-eaters and 31 546 non meat-eaters in the UK', *Public Health Nutr*, 6: 259-269.

14. Erlund, I., Koli, R., Alfthan, G. et al. (2007) 'Favourable effects of berry consumption on platelet function, blood pressure, and HDL cholesterol', *Am J Clin Nutr*, 87:323-331.

15. Field, A.E., Gillman, M.W., Rockett, H.R. and Colditz, G.A. (2003) 'Association between fruit and vegetable intake and change in body mass index among a large sample of children and adolescents in the United States', *Int J Obes*, 27:821-826.

16. George, S.M., Park, Y., Leitzmann, M.F. et al. (2009) 'Fruit and vegetable intake and risk of cancer: a prospective cohort study', *Am J Clin Nutr*, 89: 347-353.

17. Hall, J.N., Moore, S., Harper, S.B. and Lynch, J.W. (2009) 'Global variability in fruit and vegetable consumption', *Am J Prev Med*, 36: 402-409.

18. Hamer, M. and Chida, Y. (2007) 'Intake of fruit, vegetables, and antioxidants and risk of type 2 diabetes: systematic review

and meta-analysis', *J Hypertens*, 25: 2361-2369.

19. Hamidi, M., Boucher, B.A., Cheung, A.M. et al. (2011) 'Fruit and vegetable intake and bone health in women aged 45 years and over: a systematic review', *Osteoporos Int*, 22:1681-1693.

20. Harding, A.H., Wareham, N.J., Bingham, S.A. et al. (2008) 'Plasma vitamin C level, fruit and vegetable consumption, and the risk of new-onset type 2 diabetes mellitus: the European prospective investigation of cancer—Norfolk prospective study', *Arch Intern Med,* 168: 1493-1499.

21. He, F.J., Nowson, C.A. and MacGregor, G.A. (2006) 'Fruit and vegetable consumption and stroke: meta-analysis of cohort studies', *Lancet,* 367: 320-326.

22. He, F.J., Nowson, C.A., Lucas, M. and Macgregor, G.A. (2007) 'Increased consumption of fruit and vegetables is related to a reduced risk of coronary heart disease: meta-analysis of cohort studies', *J Hum Hypertens*, 21: 717-728.

23. Hoffmann, K., Boeing, H., Volatier, J.L. and Becker, W. (2003) 'Evaluating the potential health gain of the World Health Organization's recommendation concerning vegetable and fruit consumption', *Public Health Nutr*, 6: 765-772.

24. Hung, H.C., Joshipura, K.J., Jiang, R. et al. (2004) 'Fruit and vegetable intake and risk of major chronic disease', *J Natl Cancer Inst*, 96:1577-1584.

25. John, J.H., Ziebland, S., Yudkin, P. et al. (2002) 'Effects of fruit and vegetable consumption on plasma antioxidant concentrations and blood pressure: a randomised controlled trial', *Lancet,* 359:1969-1974.

26. Key, T.J. (2011) 'Fruit and vegetables and cancer risk', *Br J Cancer*, 104: 6-11.

27. Nuñez-Cordoba, J.M., Alonso, A., Beunza, J.J. et al. (2002)

'Role of vegetables and fruits in Mediterranean diets to prevent hypertension', *Eur J Clin Nutr*, 63: 605-612.

28. Riboli, E, and Norat, T. (2003) 'Epidemiologic evidence of the protective effect of fruit and vegetables on cancer risk', *Am J Clin Nutr*, 78:559S-569S.

29. Rolls, B.J., Ello-Martin, J.A. and Tohill, B.C. (2004) 'What can intervention studies tell us about the relationship between fruit and vegetable consumption and weight management?' *Nutr Rev,* 62:1-17.

30. Zino, S., Skeaff, M., Williams, S. and Mann, J. (1997) 'Randomised controlled trial of effect of fruit and vegetable consumption on plasma concentrations of lipids and antioxidants', *BMJ*, 314:1787-179.